Dr. Cimino's Weight Loss Solution

The <u>No</u> Calorie Counting

<u>No</u> Exercise

Rapid Weight Loss Plan

Scott A. Cimino, MD FACEP, FAAEM

ISBN: 978-1-0741-7002-8

Dedication

To **Jesus of Nazareth**, who taught me,

"Wisdom is vindicated by all of her daughters."

-Luke 7:35

To **Jessica, Izzy, Evey, and Sammy,**

Who remind me every day that, "The greatest things in life are free, and gifts from God are gifts indeed."

To my sister **Karen**, with whom I share a mutation in the HLA gene;

Mine resulted in Diabetes, and yours in Psoriatic Arthritis. Let's beat them both with hormones.

CONTENTS

AUTHOR'S NOTE AND DISCLAIMER

The reader should consult their personal physician before beginning any weight loss plan or changes to diet. Discuss the material presented in this book with the physician who knows you best before making any changes.

Likewise, this book is not intended to be a substitute for the professional medical care of a physician. The reader should regularly consult their physician for all health-related problems and routine care.

Section I

A Broken System

CHAPTER 1: **SOMETHING ISN'T RIGHT!**

Wake Up Call

Nearly a decade ago, I had my first wake-up call. I sat awkwardly in my chair, staring at my residency program director. It was year 2 of my emergency medicine residency, and I had been called in to discuss "a matter" with the head physician of our program. "Scott," she said gruffly, "You are too fat to ride in the helicopter."

In the second year of emergency medicine training, young resident doctors take a month to fly with the "Life-Flight" emergency medical service helicopter, helping to transport critically ill patients from the field to the hospital. Often intense and life-saving medicine is performed in and around this critical helicopter service.

"Too fat?" I stammered. Sure, I had put on a few pounds in medical school and early residency, but too fat for the helicopter? "The weight limit is 250 lbs.," She continued. "You are what they call TFTF…Too fat to fly." She went on to explain that the weight of the helicopter had to be precisely balanced, and "Also, the other crew members won't be able to move around you easily during transport."

Ouch! That Stung!

In college, I had weighed between 185 and 200 lbs, but in late medical school, I had ballooned up to 260, and through early residency even higher to 300 lbs. At a modest 5' 11", this put me at a BMI of 41 and Obesity Class III. How had it gotten this bad? With a constant cycle of studying and working odd hours to earn my medical degree and board certification, I had just never let the truth of my weight gain sink in. That is, until this moment.

From that moment on, and through the rest of the past decade, I began the process of trying to lose weight. Almost all of us are familiar with this process. I sought out and tried almost every diet known to humankind. I tracked calories until I was blue in the face. I counted "points," calculating fiber to fat ratios. I even bought pre-portioned meals. I exercised relentlessly. I read everything I could find in modern medicine that provided the "formula" for weight loss. The results were exactly what you would expect. I would lose 20-30 pounds, then be overcome by hunger, followed by indifference to weight loss, and then gain all the weight, and often more, back. Worse still, each cycle of diet, weight loss, and hunger seemed to get worse and worse and worse.

As I failed on diet after diet, I began to ask myself a question: "What are we missing?" I began to look back in history and discovered, to my amazement, almost no one was fat before the 1970s. Perhaps more importantly, many people in the 1950s and 1960s would be considered "too thin" by today's standards. The average 1950's male weighed in near the "underweight" category of our modern BMI charts, and looked down-right gaunt!

Suddenly after 1970, obesity went nuts in modern America. This piqued my interest. How could fatness be so rampant in our time, but almost non-existent in time so recent? Why were our grandparents thin, but we struggle on diet after diet, ceaselessly pounding away at the gym, barely losing any weight? Why were there no huge gym franchises in the 1950s? Why has the diet industry become a billion-dollar money-maker only in the last 40 years?

These questions kept me up at night. They pushed me to read medical research paper after research paper. I became obsessed with **what changed**. The question resounded in my mind, "Why is everyone fat?"

Before I truly understood obesity, I remember sitting at my desk in the ER, weighing 302 pounds. I sighed as my belly pushed on my scrubs, stretched nearly to bursting. I considered, briefly, taking a pair of trauma scissors and cutting the sides of my scrub top to allow room for my ever-growing girth. At that moment I looked around and took stock of our world. What I saw horrified me. My nurses were all overweight. My patients were all overweight. The clerk at the front desk of the ER was overweight. The x-ray tech was overweight. Even the paramedics bringing patients by ambulance to the ER were overweight. As I watched the next patient coming from the waiting room struggle to walk under the encumbrance of her own body, I shook my head. Something was wrong with this country. Something was wrong with this world.

Suddenly the problem became much simpler. I realized in an instant that medicine has gotten it wrong. The old model of our understanding of obesity is incomplete and willfully simplistic. Modern medicine, in its arrogance, hasn't noticed that an entire generation has gotten fat without an adequate explanation. We are not eating too much and exercising too little; rather, we are doing something differently than our grandparents and great-grandparents did. We are doing something differently than all of our ancestors throughout all of time, and it is making us fat! Our mission should be to find what that difference is.

In my current practice, I spend almost every day treating patients who suffer from diseases that are completely avoidable. Nearly every patient I see takes medication for high blood pressure, high cholesterol, and diabetes. Almost all of them are overweight or obese. Most of them think they are failures and beyond hope. As a young physician, I believed the teachings of modern medicine. I thought these patients simply ate too much and exercised too little. I fully endorsed the idea that they were lazy and gluttonous. I judged them, and myself, for a failure that was not their own. Can you blame a person for being poisoned? Or for following bad advice? Our generation has been lied to and poisoned almost since birth.

Besides working as a physician, I am also a type 1 diabetic. I was diagnosed with the disease at age 9. Likely you or someone you know has diabetes. In both types 1 and 2 of diabetes, there is inadequate control of your body's blood glucose.

Throughout my life and medical training, I have had to manage blood glucose levels endlessly, often at the most inopportune times. It was not uncommon during busy shifts in the ER to have to stop examining a patient to check my blood glucose or to eat a piece of candy, only to return when I had corrected my own body. Diabetes is a constant roller-coaster between high and low blood glucose levels. Low blood glucose makes you feel nauseated, irritable, shaky, sweaty, and extremely fatigued. High blood glucose makes you feel tired, groggy, nauseous, and sluggish.

Because of this, for a long time, I viewed my diabetes as a curse. In type 1 (my type), the diabetic must take injections of insulin to compensate for the destruction of vital pancreas cells. Prior to the 1920s, type 1 diabetes was a fatal diagnosis for children. But, as fate would have it, it turns out that insulin plays a vital role in why we are fat.

Because of the vital role of insulin in obesity, I now view my type 1 diabetes as a blessing, rather than a curse. Type 1 diabetes has offered me a unique window into the inner workings of the human body. I am in direct control of my body's insulin levels. I take near-constant blood glucose readings to control my disease. Though this is frustrating and often very annoying, it has provided me with an insight I would not trade for anything in the world.

As you will see throughout this book, the very key to our weight is our insulin. By managing my insulin, as I will teach you to do, I have found the formula to lose weight effortlessly. As a physician and a type 1 diabetic, I am in a unique position to evaluate each food's effect on our internal hormones. In other words, I can experiment on myself and report those findings to you.

In this book, my goal is to teach you to reboot your system and change the hormonal state of your body. Instead of eating less and exercising more, our goal will be to change how you eat to make you similar to a human being in the 1960s. We are going to try to take you back to a time in which humans thought more about life and less about being fat. By rebooting your hormones, you will simply melt down to your ideal body weight. So much so that I even considered calling this program "the melt diet."

This book is the summation of all that I have learned and all of my experimentation. By following the rules which I will outline in this book, I have lost 116 lbs. I currently weigh 186 lbs., down from a starting point of 302 lbs. I do not struggle to maintain my weight. I never feel "starving" or tired. My diabetic blood glucose control is near-perfect. It is, in a word, easy. What's more, after implementing this plan, I was able to reach my goal weight in about six months. That is an average weight loss of 5 lbs. per week, and ridiculous by normal dieting standards.

Further yet, because I totally reject the teachings of modern medicine on obesity and nutrition, I wanted to prove that our obesity epidemic has nothing to do with lack of exercise. I insisted that my new approach to obesity be done *without* exercise, as I did not want to design and prove yet another "eat nothing, exercise more" program.

Throughout my entire 116 lb. weight loss, I did not do one single exercise. I never went to the gym. I never lifted weights. I never ran. I never even took walks. Is exercise bad? Certainly not! I am certain, had I exercised even lightly, my weight loss would have been even more rapid. But that is not the point. The point is that America is putting the wrong sort of fuel into the engine of our body, and if we fix the fuel, we fix obesity. For this reason, I chose not to exercise: not because it is bad, but because it is not the problem.

As we go forward in the coming chapters, we will explore the major changes to the American diet, which have happened since the 1960s. As you learn these changes, you will begin to understand how we have gone off course and hijacked our body's systems to be increasingly obese. After this, we will look at our body's hormonal system. Finally, we will create a system of rules which will cause your body to rid itself of excess fat.

This weight loss program is for anyone who feels like there is no answer. This was written for anyone who feels like every expert is wrong, and that there is simply no way to lose weight. I know, because I was that person. If you are tired of following each fad diet or calorie tracking program, only to fall back into fatness after months of hunger and grumpiness, I understand. I was there. But this program is not that. This program is about taking back control of your body's own hormones. These hormones were given to you by God to help you naturally maintain your weight. And we are going to use them again!

Some of the teachings in this book may seem difficult at first. But I ask you to trust me. They are not difficult, but rather new and different. If you will not trust me, then trust my weight loss. It works.

If you will try the principles in this book, I will make you several promises. The first promise is this: On diets which make you count calories or track "points," you become increasingly hungry until you give up. On this program, your hunger will decrease until you are almost always disinterested in food. Second, you will not experience the normal irritability, tiredness, and grumpiness associated with other diets. Rather on this program, you will have increased energy and at times, even euphoria. Third, I promise you will laugh at how you used to struggle with weight, and how ridiculously simple it is to be thin once you understand your body.

So, for all of you who are fed up with being fat; for all of you who are tired of your doctor's raised eyebrows and condescension; for all of you who think there is simply no way to get thin, welcome to the Dr. Cimino Weight Loss Solution. This is for you.

CHAPTER 2: **THE WORLD GOT FAT!**

Look Around!

The next time that you go out into public, I want you to take inventory of your fellow human beings. Look around at the people in today's world, hustling, and bustling, driving to work, buying things at the store, living their lives. Get out of your mental bubble and truly look at your neighbors. How do they look? Do they look healthy and well?

What you will find are a generation of overweight, often obese individuals and children. You will see dark circles under eyes, sallow skin, and tired expressions. Most are on antidepressants or anti-anxiety medications. Almost all are overweight. Many are dangerously so. Stress is rampant.

Now let's take it a step further. Let's count them. Not the fat people. That would be far too easy. The next time you are in public, I want you to count the thin people. Take stock and honestly count how many people you see who are "at goal weight." Count the folks who truly seem to have their weight under control - the people who look healthy. You won't get very high. America's obesity epidemic is booming at an alarming rate. But why?

In America today, nearly 1 out of every 2 individuals is obese. The CDC reports 39.6% of all American adults rank in the obese classification. In the age group of 40-60, this number is even higher at 42.8%. This is staggering. For every two people you know, one of them is putting their health at tremendous risk due to the amount of excess and unnecessary fat on their body.

But what about the other person? The other 1 out of 2? Are we to assume that the other half of Americans, therefore, are thin? Far from it. If we include the category of "overweight," which is just shy of Obesity Class 1, 71.6% of Americans are included. This means that almost all of us are carrying excess weight, increasing our risk of disease and early death. What has happened?

Recently at the grocery store, I performed this mental exercise. As a physician, my heart was saddened. Out of 50 unique individuals I observed, I counted only five individuals I would consider "at goal weight." 5 out of 50! After shaking my head in disbelief, I wondered to myself what it would be like to walk around a 1960s grocery store. How would my count have been then? I don't have a time machine. But, luckily, we have the data.

In the 1960s, the average US human being was thin. Sure, there was the occasional husky adult or even teenager, but by and large, people were trim. Think back to pictures of your grandparents or great-grandparents. For most of you, this memory will include pictures of people who look like the extreme dieters of today's generation – the fitness freaks that hit the gym 24/7 in the modern world and yet still struggle to keep weight off.

Here is a picture of my wife's grandparents in 1950:

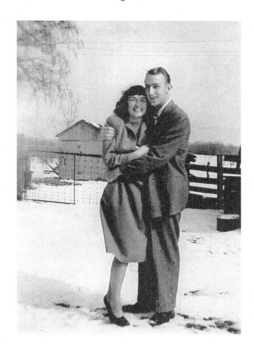

That is a trim couple! Did they hit the gym every morning at 5 AM? Did they constantly think about their diet? Of course not! Grandpa Harry went to work, came home and had a steak dinner followed by a stiff drink, then went to bed. No gym, no calorie tracking, just life! In fact, "gyms" barely existed!

Up until the 1970s that was just the norm. According to a CDC study spanning the four decades from 1960 to 2002, the average weight for Americans has sky-rocketed despite an increase in dieting and time spent exercising. In 1960 the average male weighed in at 166.3 lbs. Very svelte, indeed! As of 2016, the average American male weighed 197.8 pounds (89.7 kg), ranking in the "obese" classification. And remember, averages don't represent the true picture. Averages include the underweight, as well as all age groups. From my medical practice, the average 20 to 40-year-old male I see in the office has a weight of around 225 pounds (102 kg).

Despite getting fatter, the average time spent exercising, on the other hand, has increased. Today the average weekly time spent at the gym, or doing aerobic exercise, is 2 hours. In 1960, the average time spent devoted to exercise was next to 0.

Many physicians today would have you believe we are a "lazier generation." Somehow, they believe the American's of the 1960s walked more, and we less. Do they realize they had cars in the 1960s? Do they realize that Gold's Gym, LA Fitness, and 24-Hour Fitness did not yet exist? Indeed, there were almost no gyms whatsoever. The popular franchise gyms were invented in the late 1970s and 1980s, very much in response to a growing obesity epidemic. If they were a response to a problem, they could not also be the source of the problem. In truth, today, we are the most aggressive exercisers in human history. There is just one problem: exercise isn't the issue!

The average woman in 1960 was likewise a healthy 140.2 pounds (63.7 kg). While height has stayed the same, the average female weight has since ballooned to 170.5 pounds (77.5 kg) in 2016, again in the obese designation. This has increased by nearly 10 pounds since 2000 when the average female weight was 163 pounds. Only God knows what our weights will be in 2020, 2025, or 2030.

Children have not been spared by this American crisis, either. The average weight for a 10-year-old boy in 1963 was 74.2 pounds (33.7 kg). Today that average has increased by roughly 10% to 85 pounds (38.6 kg). 10-year-old girls faired roughly the same, increasing from 77.4 pounds (35.2 kg) to 88 pounds (40 kg) in 2002.

As you can see, America is getting significantly fatter. Look around at your friends, family, and even yourself. The data tells us that at least 1 out of every 2 people you know is obese. 3 out of every 4 are overweight. Do these statistics fit the picture? I think they do. Now pretend you live in the 1960s. In your mind, look around at all of your friends, family, and coworkers. During this era before our obesity epidemic, it would have required you to count 20 people before you found a fat one. The difference is alarming.

Obesity Worldwide

Prior to 2000, many nations in the world laughed at the "fat Americans" and our obesity crisis. Almost none of them are laughing now. Obesity has spread like a plague throughout the entire world. Even cultures we once regarded as staples of thinness, such as Japan and China, are beginning to see rapidly rising obesity.

China, in particular, now has a population with type 2 diabetes and obesity, which is greater than the *entire population of Australia*, and rivals our own obese population in America. The current prevalence of type 2 diabetes in China is 9.7%, just edging out the United States, where diabetes prevalence stands at 9.4%. At a population of 1 billion, that is a lot of diabetics! Type 2 diabetes, a common complication of obesity, has increased in China from 1994, at which time only 2.5% of the population was diabetic. Something has happened to cause this upsurge, but the "why" remains a mystery. In China today, the business of gastric bypass, or obesity surgery, is exploding!

Likewise, in Japan, obesity is soaring. Parents are getting gastric bypass surgery for children as young as five years old. Today, over half of the obese children in the world live in Asia.

The United Kingdom, likewise, has seen a dramatic increase in obesity over the last 20 years. Low-income industrial areas have been hit worst by the growing epidemic. In 1966 the proportion of people in the United Kingdom with a BMI over 30 (obese) was a meager 1.2% for men and 1.8% for women. That is less than 1 out of 50. By 1989 these figures had risen to 10.6% for men and 14.0% for women. Today, the numbers stand at 35.1% of adults obese, with 17% of children aged 2-15 similarly affected. In 50 years, obesity has increased by 3,500%! What the heck is going on?

Even the once lean French, often credited with their trim walking-intense lifestyles have begun to succumb to some unseen force driving fatness worldwide.

But by far, the greatest rises in obesity are in the developing nations of the world. In Africa, the number of obese children under five years of age has increased by 50% since 2000. Where 1 out of 9 children in Africa suffers from malnourishment, today, 1 out of 10 children in Africa now suffers from obesity. By 2022, it is expected the number of obese children in Africa will outpace the number of undernourished.

Ethiopia, often seen as a land stricken by hunger, has seen an increase in obese women to rates 600% percent higher than in the year 2004.

As I mentioned, the world is no longer laughing at American obesity. Whatever the cause may be, it has spread. Like a disease, fatness is consuming whole populations. This unknown obesity-causer is spreading out its tendrils into every nation and people.

It may surprise you to learn that America is not the fattest nation on earth. We are surpassed by:

10 MOST OBESE NATIONS

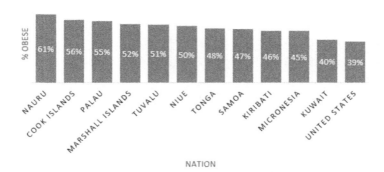

Nauru, the Fattest Place on Earth

The leader of this list is Nauru, the fattest place on earth. Nauru is a small Pacific island. In time immemorial, the Nauru people were fit and healthy. They lived off of the land, actively fishing, growing, and harvesting. In 1914, the Nauru were muscular and trim.

Throughout the 1900s, the Nauru people grew temporarily

wealthy through the discovery of precious minerals on their island. This allowed them to import food, rather than harvest it from their land. The imported food, because it had to travel such far distances, was processed rather than locally grown or gathered. Increases in obesity began almost immediately.

Later, their mineral mines failed. The temporarily wealth ended, but the Nauru people had a problem. They could no longer remember the natural fishing and gathering ways of their ancestors, and so they continued to lean on imported processed foods. Today the Nauru people have an obesity rate of 61% of the general population, with almost 100% overweight.

The alteration of the Nauru diet was the single greatest change to their society in their entire history. Yet still, people insist their obesity epidemic is only because they are "lazier" than in prior generations. Ridiculous!

Even Our Thin are Fat

At least we aren't as fat as the nine countries above us, right? Not so fast. There is another way to be fat in America, even if the chart calls you normal weight. This problem is seldom discussed in modern medicine, but when it was discovered, its significance shocked the medical community. The problem is known colloquially as "TOFI." It stands for "Thin Outside, Fat Inside."

The idea is that a person can look reasonably thin on the outside, where external fat normally gathers, yet still harbor dangerous visceral fat around their organs. Their misleading external appearance leads their doctors and health professionals, as well as their loved ones, to assume they are healthy. However, when they are run through imaging techniques (such as MRI or x-ray absorptiometry), we see an entirely different picture. Radiographic imaging reveals "fat insides." Their organs are coated in thick layers of visceral fat.

In 2014, a study was performed to evaluate visceral fat or TOFI. In the study, X-ray absorptiometry imaging was performed on 12,217 individuals over age 20. The findings were remarkable. Of the "normal weight" people imaged during the study, a whopping 32% had internal fat at levels which would, if the BMI chart were more accurate, rank them as overweight or even obese. Visceral obesity is a serious health risk. All studies done on obesity have shown that visceral fat is the most dangerous type of fat. It is this fat which is most closely linked to type 2 diabetes, as well as a myriad of other complications. And at least one-third of our thin people have it! If these individuals were included in our weight statistics, our rate of overweight Americans would be well above 85%.

"TOFI" also explains the phenomenon of the thin, healthy-appearing individual in America who is suddenly told they have type 2 diabetes, high blood pressure, or any number of other weight-related diseases, all while appearing perfectly thin.

But the take away from "TOFI" is much more significant. What "TOFI" means is that whatever the cause of obesity in America may be, the culprit is so toxic, so insidious, that it can disease even someone who works out relentlessly, diets relentlessly, and, by all modern measurements, appears healthy.

Something Has Changed, But What?

Undoubtedly, something has changed since the era of the 1960s, as well as all-time before. Today many blame portion size, or lack of exercise. But what if the true answer is more complex? What if something we are doing is changing our metabolic rate? Luckily, past research can give us some clues into the metabolisms of the past.

Between November 19th, 1944, and December 20th, 1945, the famous Minnesota Experiment was performed. The experiment sought to understand the effects of starvation. The participants in the trial, 25-year-old men, were "conscientious" objectors to World War II. Because of their objection to serving in the war, they were "encouraged" to volunteer for human experimentation instead. Indeed, this was a different time.

In the study, the men began at very normal and healthy weights. During a 12-week control period, they were fed a daily 3200 calories, with the goal of maintaining their weight under observation. Today, 3200 calories would be considered an aggressive weight-gain diet, yet most of the participants maintained their weight on 3200 calories, and some even lost weight. None gained.

During the following six months, the participants were placed on a "starvation" calorie regimen of 1,560 calories. Today, 1500 calories is the typical weight-loss regimen often recommended by doctors. Since we follow this dietary advice of 1500 calories for weight loss today, you would expect the men of the 1940s slowly lost weight, as we do, on this diet. Right?

But that assumption would be wrong. Over the next six months, on 1,560 calories, the men of the Minnesota experiment nearly starved to death.

During the course of the experiment, the men became sickly thin. They thought about food constantly. They dreamed about food. They talked incessantly about food. They had food-related psychosis, hallucinating about food.

How can today's generation use 1500 calories as the safe recommendation for weight loss dieting, yet in the 1940s the same calories nearly killed a group of young men? The answer is that their metabolisms were much, much higher.

Working backward from the data, we can extrapolate the men's starting metabolisms by how much weight they lost after beginning this calorie restriction diet. It turns out their resting basal metabolic rates were roughly 3500 to 4000 calories per day. This is more than double the currently recognized metabolism of a modern man. Today we recognize the average male metabolism at 1800 calories per day. How then, may you ask, can the literal halving of the average male metabolism be explained? This is an excellent question and the goal of this book!

Obesity: The Cause of Almost Every Modern Disease

Both the obese in America, as well as the "TOFI" Americans,

suffer similar fates as their life progresses. They go on to develop a very predictable pattern of diseases which, unfortunately, are never discussed between physician and patient as all stemming from the same source: obesity. In modern medicine, we call the pattern of developing several diseases, all of which stem from excess body fat, "Metabolic Syndrome."

The classic metabolic syndrome consists of Hypertension (high blood pressure), Diabetes (insulin resistance and elevated blood glucose), Hypercholesterolemia (High Cholesterol), and increased abdominal and visceral body fat. These diseases increase the risk of cardiovascular disease and death, as well as stroke.

Physicians began to notice this pattern in the early 1900s. In 1923 a Swedish physician named Kylin described a nebulous picture of a human being with high blood pressure, high blood sugar, and high uric acid levels (leading to gout). Later in 1947, the French clinician Vague tied these diseases to fat distribution throughout the body, associating them with visceral obesity.

By 1988 an American endocrinologist named Gerry Reaven gave the now-famous "Banting Lecture," in which he described "Syndrome X," "a cluster of risk factors for diabetes and cardiovascular disease." His contribution was monumental, adding, for the first time, the concept that a human may become resistant to his or her own hormones, namely insulin.

Following Reaven's findings, in 1992 the term "Insulin Resistance Syndrome" was tried, but was quickly replaced with today's terminology. Today it is widely called Metabolic Syndrome.

Unfortunately for Americans today, Metabolic Syndrome does not go far enough to describe the true picture of an obese or inwardly fat (TOFI) human being's disease pattern. There are many other diseases caused by obesity, most of which you will never hear your physician link to your weight. But as more and more research is done, it is becoming crystal clear that almost every modern disease stems from excess body fat and insulin resistance. Modern medicine knows how to treat pneumonia, skin infections, tuberculosis, and almost all of the diseases which plagued our ancestors. We are incapable, however, of addressing all of the diseases of diet which have reared their heads in our time.

Some of the biggest offenders of obesity-induced disease, rarely discussed, include autoimmune and inflammatory diseases, joint and musculoskeletal disease, sleep apnea, fertility issues, and sex hormone imbalances.

1. Autoimmune/Inflammatory – Excess body fat is highly inflammatory. Study after study shows a link between obesity and autoimmune diseases such as Crohn's, Ulcerative Colitis, Psoriasis, Rheumatism, and a host of others.

2. Joint and Musculoskeletal – Perhaps unsurprisingly, chronic back problems and chronic joint problems (most commonly knee) are due to the overloading of a skeleton built for 140-160 pounds carrying 100 lbs. of extra weight day-in, day-out.

3. Sleep Apnea – Sleep apnea is a condition in which a person will cease breathing several times throughout the night. What physicians will not tell you is that this is almost always caused by excess fat in the airway. This excess fat stops airflow into the trachea when the neck is relaxed in sleep. This leads to right-sided heart failure and is traditionally treated with a C-PAP machine worn during sleep. In greater than 90% of cases, this disease will disappear with as little as 30 pounds of weight loss.

4. Infertility and Polycystic Ovarian Syndrome – Today, many women are diagnosed with Polycystic Ovarian Syndrome (formerly Polycystic Ovarian Disease). They are told their ovaries make cysts, impeding fertility, and that they must be treated with hormone shots to enable pregnancy. But did you know that if you are a woman, excess fat continually converts your estrogen into testosterone?

The entire issue of fertility stems from this conversion of estrogen to testosterone. In medical school, we are taught that obese women, at higher testosterone levels than their thin peers, often have hairier arms and upper lips. The excess testosterone, besides causing unwanted hair growth, is causing infertility, and yet their physicians often don't have the courage to tell them, "this is all your weight!"

5.   Low T – Men suffer a similar fate. Today, men are in a craze over "Low T," which stands for Low Testosterone. They often take monthly intra-muscular pellets or shots to increase testosterone levels. What is often neglected, however, is the fact that their excess fat is stealing their testosterone and converting it to estrogen! This leads to anxiety, depression, decreased fertility, gynecomastia (male breasts), and decreased energy.

What Is Going On?

Almost no physician today will dispute the fact that obesity is a rising problem in the United States, as well as the world. Similarly, almost no physician would argue that the bulk of diseases which we physicians treat are related to weight. On obesity, the argument in medicine is not over whether we are getting fatter, but rather why.

I stand firmly opposed to physicians and scientists, no matter their credentials in endocrinology, public health, or nutrition, who argue that this generation simply eats too much. If this were true, what would be the explanation for why we eat too much after millennia of maintaining our weight? Why then doesn't calorie restriction dieting work long-term? Why is obesity spreading from nation to nation? Isn't it more likely, something we are eating is causing this new pandemic?

In addressing the spreading obesity, we must look at it like any other disease. Something, like a poison, is destroying our body's ability to maintain our weight. This something is spreading across the world rapidly. Our goal is to find out what it is.

Did the human body change in 40-50 years? Did our core genetics deteriorate? Have we evolved into a different sluggishly fat species, unable to control our appetites? Did our fundamental DNA change? Of course not! The difference must be purely external!

If our ancestors were effortlessly thin, and we are effortlessly fat, something is to blame. Generally, we blame ourselves and each other. But is it believable that every generation prior to ours had more willpower and self-control? Is it believable that lions, tigers, bears, zebras, giraffes, and all other creatures on God's earth know how to maintain their weight automatically, but humans in the last 50 years don't?

To date, the explanation of modern medicine is inadequate. Next, let's take a look at what your physician was taught about our growing obesity crisis.

CHAPTER 3: **THE TWO THEORIES OF OBESITY**

A Little Secret

I'm going to let you in on a little secret about physicians. This secret is not commonly acknowledged, nor is it discussed openly within medical circles. The secret is this: Doctors don't know anything about nutrition or weight loss. That's right. *Nothing*. After 12 years of training in college, medical school, and residency, we don't know a darn thing. We are woefully unprepared to face a generation of morbidly obese, diabetic, and dying patients. We are sadly ignorant of the true origin of obesity in those we seek to help. This lack of knowledge leads us to prescribe medicines to treat the symptoms of a problem, rather than to cure the problem itself.

The reason for this lack of knowledge is tied back to our training. In medical school, we are taught very little about weight gain and weight maintenance. Our training, by and large, comes from the standard wisdom disseminated throughout the last 50 years by the Department of Agriculture, American Medical Association, American Heart Association, and other entities which presume to understand the science of obesity.

Obesity today is the leading cause of disease and death in America, yet your physician learned a model for the pathology of weight gain, which is the scientific equivalent of a finger-painting. During a stunningly short 2-hour lecture on the subject, we are told that the "Calories Eaten – Calories Burned = Body Fat." In other words, "Eat too much, get fat. Eat too little, get thin." That's it. That's all. Next subject!

The Simplistic Model of Obesity

The "Calories In - Calories Out" model is the pervading theory of obesity. It is a theory which dictates that any calories your body takes in, which you subsequently do not burn, are stored as fat. So simple! I'm glad we figured that out so quickly!

This theory often cites Newton's First Law of Thermodynamics to prove its point. The First Law of Thermodynamics states, "Energy and Matter can neither be created nor destroyed." On this law of physics, I think we can all agree. However, when applied to the energy balance and fat storage of a human being, things get tricky.

Modern nutrition science applies this first law of thermodynamics to the human body, stating, "Calories eaten that are not burned as energy, cannot otherwise be destroyed, and thus are stored as fat." This is wildly simplistic. Because of the simplistic nature of this understanding of obesity, the advice given by the medical community is equally simple: Eat Less and Exercise More.

To decrease the number of calories you store as fat, modern physicians and nutritionists advise you to reduce how many calories you eat each day, while simultaneously increasing your physical exertion. This, they believe, will result in a negative energy balance, forcing your body to utilize fat for fuel and subsequently lose weight.

The USDA puts it this way "Reaching a healthier weight is a balancing act. The secret is learning how to balance your energy in and energy out", and further "Weight loss can be achieved either by eating fewer calories or by burning more calories with physical activity, preferably both."

The CDC advises the following on weight loss: "If you take in more calories than you use, you will still gain weight…If you need to gain or lose weight, you'll need to balance your diet and activity level to achieve your goal."

The American Medical Association states, "If you are gaining weight, you are eating too many calories. If your weight is stable, you know that this many calories works for weight maintenance. But you will need to decrease your calorie intake to lose weight."

You can see that these people all learned exactly what your physician was taught in medical school. Eat less, exercise more. So simple. There is only one problem: *It doesn't work!* This is precisely what modern medical schools teach. It is what modern nutritionists truly believe. And it is dead wrong.

The Dismal Data on "Eat Less, Exercise More"

If you follow your doctor's advice, you will restrict your calories down to 1500, or possibly 1200 per day. You will simultaneously begin doing new exercises. Perhaps you will begin walking or running daily in an effort to burn an extra 200 calories. Perhaps you will buy an aerobics video and begin religiously lifting your knees in your living room throughout the early morning. You will reduce fat, weigh your food, and say ridiculous things like "Can you take the skin off my chicken breast?"

Will you lose weight? Yes, you will. And you will do so for the exact reason that modern physicians and nutritionists say: Your calories burned will exceed your calories taken in. But there is just one problem. Your weight will fall for about 3 to 4 months, but after this time period, your weight loss will stop. You will be overcome with hunger and fatigue. Your metabolism will come to a screeching halt. You will give up, stop all exercise and dieting, and your weight will balloon upward, often exceeding the weight you held before beginning this fruitless program.

How do I know this will happen? Because every study performed on "Eat Less, Exercise More" weight loss programs show it to be true. The estimated failure rate of this type of diet program is close to 99%.

In a 2010 study, Only 1 in 6 overweight adults in the US maintained weight loss of at least 10% for one year or longer. At 250 pounds, this would represent an initial 25-pound weight loss. After one year, that 25 pounds was regained in 83% of individuals. After two years, the weight was regained by nearly 100% of participants.

In the Women's Health Initiative Study, nearly 50,000 women were recruited to study dietary effects on weight loss and cardiac health. This study, one of the most massive, well-funded, and overall impressive studies on "eat less exercise more" ever performed followed women for 7.5 years. The control group did not adjust diet or exercise at all, while the intervention group reduced calories from roughly 1800 calories per day to 1450 calories per day (a drop of 350 calories per day).

The expected weight loss from the calorie reduction alone would be 1 pound every 10 days, or 36.5 pounds per year. This doesn't even count exercise! The women continued this calorie reduction for 7.5 years. What do you think happened? If we follow the simplistic model of obesity, these women should have been vastly underweight by the 7.5-year follow-up. After 7.5 years, however, the group who exercised and reduced calories weighed only 2.2 pounds less than the group which did neither.

That's right, 7.5 years of reduced calories and increased exercise, with a resulting 2.2 pounds of weight loss. How sad!

In another large study, 5,145 overweight and obese adults with type 2 diabetes began an intensive program to educate and encourage weight loss. Participants were given counseling, and during the first six months, they reduced calories substantially and increased exercise to 3 hours per week. They were then followed for eight years. Throughout the subsequent eight years, they continued dietary and exercise goals.

At eight years, the mean weight loss was 4.7%. For a 250-pound man, this means after eight years of trying to obtain normal weight, they lost only 12 pounds. That is just over 1 pound per year. Even in their most successful participants, who lost 10% or higher, this would only equate to a 25-pound weight loss over eight years or 3 pounds per year. I don't know about you, but if I am only losing 3 pounds per year, I am giving up!

But this result is not uncommon. In a 2005 review of 33 clinical trials involving weight loss with diet and exercise, ranging from 10 weeks to 1 year, the review found that almost half of the initial weight loss achieved in a calorie-restriction diet was regained at a 1 year follow up. When we follow up at further dates, as was done in the Women's Health Initiative, we see that almost 100% of the weight is regained, despite faithfulness to the program.

Often the poor results of "Eat Less, Exercise More" diets are so dismal that researchers categorize success as maintaining a 5% weight loss at 1-2 years. If you are a 200-pound woman, this means *success* is keeping 10 pounds off. No one, including yourself, should consider this success. Success is obtaining **normal weight**.

What Happens at 4 Months?

Why is the 4-month point in an "Eat Less, Exercise More" diet so important? Why do so many diets fail at this point? The answer is surprisingly simple. After eating less and exercising more, your body senses that you are in a net calorie deficit. Because of this deficit, the body *slows your metabolism*. This process of slowing the metabolism takes, on average, about 4 months.

Think of this like a household budget. Your body, over the course of 4 months, notices that the household has suddenly stopped earning as much money (calories). Simultaneously, it has begun spending money on things like new furniture and jewelry (New exercise routine). After about 4 months of this activity, the head of household (the hypothalamus) puts its foot down. "It's time to tighten the budget!" In terms of the hypothalamus, tightening the budget equates to lowering the basal metabolism.

For the first few months of your new "Eat Less, Exercise More" routine, your body has not yet slowed its metabolism. But at the 4-month point, the body has slowly reduced your calorie expenditure to match your new diet and exercise routine. The household budget now matches the household income. The result is a calorie deficit of zero and stalled weight loss. Worse, you are now in a dangerous situation. If you stop exercising or begin eating even a little bit more food each day, you will gain the weight back!

Though things are balanced, the body hates persisting at a reduced caloric rate. While slowing your metabolism, the body tries desperately to encourage you to begin eating like you previously did.

In a 2011 study, researchers enrolled 50 overweight or obese patients in a 10-week weight loss program in which very low calories were prescribed. After 10 weeks of calorie restriction, the researchers then tested the blood levels of hormones which control hunger. They found Ghrelin, the hormone most closely linked to the hunger impulse, was present at much higher levels after the calorie reduction diet. Peptide YY, Amylin, Cholecystokinin, which are *potent inhibitors of hunger*, were found to be much lower. By month 4, the body has increased your "hunger" hormones, trying to get you to give up and eat more.

To fight your calorie restriction attempts, your hunger hormones begin to surge, increasing your drive to "raid the fridge." This feeling grows stronger and stronger until, at long last, the diet is over.

When you finally give up on your diet and exercise routine, your metabolism has slowed to a fraction of where it was before you began. The average dieter, happy to be free of the shackles of their diet, typically enjoys a very rich and satisfying bender of high-calorie foods after giving up. It is not uncommon, after quitting a diet, to enjoy a wild week of eating, consuming pizza and fast food to the tune of 4000 calories per day. In such a scenario, the dieter has the capacity to gain 7 pounds back in a single week! So much for all of your hard work.

In a 2008 study, researchers studied the changes in metabolism which occur when a person undergoes a calorie-restriction diet. A significant decrease in metabolic rate was seen in study participants beginning at a 5-10% reduction in weight. This means that a 250-pound man will slow his metabolism after losing between 12 - 25 pounds. This is when the diet really gets tough. On most weight loss programs, with an average weight loss of 1.5-pounds per week, this metabolic slowing would occur at roughly 4 months.

And worse yet, it takes time for your metabolism and hunger hormones to return to where they were before the diet, if they ever do. One study showed it can take many years for the metabolic rate to heal to its original rate after performing a calorie-restrictive diet. The study found that even over a year after the diet, (an original diet of only 8 weeks), a 10% reduction in basal metabolic rate and thermic effect of feeding were still present. The researchers commented, "Declines in energy expenditure *favoring the regain of lost weight* persist well beyond the period of dynamic weight loss." In some participants, they noted a 300 to 400 calorie difference from the control group, who did not participate in the original diet.

The same study further noted that hunger hormones at 62 weeks (just over a year), remained high, while "fullness hormones" remained startlingly low. This means that even a year after an 8-week calorie reduction diet, your hunger remains increased. With a slower metabolism and greater hunger, you are set up to gain even more weight. You would have been better off to have never dieted!

The Not-So-Subtle Implication

And to compound problems, the failed advice given by your doctor comes with a generous side serving of guilt. The inherent assumption built into the advice of "Eat Less Exercise More" is very dangerous. Lying just below the surface of this theory rests the not-so-subtle implication that anyone who is overweight is either gluttonous or lazy or both.

Obesity, to the modern physician, represents a personal failure to maintain energy balance. Overeating and too little exercise lead to fatness.

But no one chooses to be obese. Being vastly overweight comes with social ridicule, feelings of failure and inadequacy, difficulties in relationships, symptoms of joint pain, tiredness, diabetes, heart disease, increased risk of cancer, and a myriad of other issues. There is no perceptible benefit to being grossly overweight. An obese person has everything to gain by losing weight and nothing (except pounds and pants size) to lose. So, are they simply too weak to say no to the doughnut? To the pizza? As someone who was vastly overweight myself, I find this extremely insulting.

The truth is that the obese population in America has incredibly high willpower. It is not unusual to see a vastly overweight individual do extreme things to lose weight. Many of my overweight friends, myself included, have done difficult things like a 1-month juice fast, reduction of our dietary intake to 1000 calories per day, and exercising 2 hours daily at the gym. None of these, however, seem sustainable. And worse, these mechanisms of weight loss cause profound slowing of the metabolism and increased hunger. The slowed metabolism results in diminishing returns until the dieter's weight loss creeps down to nothing, and they eventually give up.

With failure rates of 99%, as well as the impossibility of overcoming a diet designed to slow your metabolism into the ground, modern physicians border on cruelty in their treatment. On the one hand, they give impossible and terrible advice, and in the next breath, they blame their patients for failure.

Often these patients redouble their efforts when the weight loss stalls out. In an effort to comply with their physician, they cut calories further, increase their exercise routine, and, for a while, lose more weight. Yet the cycle continues. In a month or so, their metabolic rate has slowed again, and they are back in the office trying to discuss a stalling weight loss with a physician who views them as weak, or worse, as a liar.

This is the great irony of our modern era. In a time when everyone is obese, no one blames the changes to our food. No one looks for an answer on what might have changed since the 1960s, a time when all humans were naturally thin. Instead, we blame the obese patient. After all, a calorie is a calorie, right? Obesity is just too many calories in, and too few calories burned, right?

It's So Simple! But Why Doesn't It Work?

If losing weight is as simple as "Eat Less, Exercise More," why doesn't it work? Why can't the average American keep weight off for more than 6 months? Why do 99% of diets fail after one year? The answer is that the simplistic model of "Eat Less, Exercise More" ignores more than 100 years of research which clearly shows that bodyweight is controlled not by calories eaten and energy expended, but rather by hormones.

As our current recommendations have failed, many physicians are beginning to look for a more complex and complete model of the cause of obesity, as well as the failure of modern weight loss programs. For this reason, a second model of obesity has been proposed. In this second model of obesity, which we will explore throughout this book, our goal is to recognize and integrate the hormonal control which the body exerts over energy balance and weight. Rather than Calories In – Calories Out, the model looks more like this:

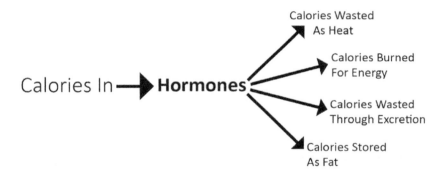

Evidence for Other Causes of Obesity

The hormonal theory of obesity did not come about randomly. In order to truly understand obesity, the more clever scientists throughout the ages have recognized that we must first evaluate some strange conditions in medicine in which weight regulation breaks down. To understand the body, it is often most helpful to study the times in which it fails to function normally.

Since the 1800s, researchers began to theorize that the hypothalamus, through hormonal input, ultimately decides body weight. By studying animals and humans in whom the hypothalamus has been injured, much has been learned about our body's natural weight control.

Patients who have suffered a traumatic brain injury, for example, sometimes sustain damage to areas of their hypothalamus. The hypothalamus is a sort of "Central Command" for hormonal direction, located in the brain. Subsequent to this hypothalamic injury, patients who have existed at a normal weight for decades have been seen to gain 150 pounds in a single year!

These individuals begin gaining weight almost immediately after their brain injury. Family and friends are often stunned. A person with no weight issues whatsoever becomes morbidly obese, almost in the blink of an eye. When these patients seek out their physician for help, they are often given the same ridiculous advice to eat less and exercise more, with disregard for their recent injury. In an effort to slow weight gain, the physicians often reduce calories to ridiculously low levels. Sometimes as few as 500 calories per day!

But since the issue is not with calories, but rather with hormonal control within the brain, what happens after these individuals decrease calories to 500 per day while simultaneously increasing exercise, as their doctors instruct them? The patients still gain body fat! That's right, despite eating a diet of 500 calories per day, these human beings, because of an injury to the hormonal control center, are still able to gain body fat. Something important is going on here.

In contrast, researchers have noted that type 1 diabetic patients, in whom the beta cells of the pancreas have been destroyed by their own immune system, lose weight at an unprecedented rate before treatment begins. Sometimes undiagnosed type 1 diabetics report losing as much as 12 pounds in a single week. That is almost 2 pounds per day. More fascinating still, these patients have been noted to lose such dramatic amounts of weight even while eating diets as high as 7,000 calories per day. The rabbit hole gets stranger!

Think about what this means: we have cases in which an

individual can eat as few as 500 calories per day and still gain body fat, and another medical condition in which a patient can eat as many as 7,000 calories per day and burn 2 pounds of body fat per day. But wait a minute, I thought it was simply "Calories In – Calories Out"?

What these examples teach us is that the calories we eat are not simply stored if we eat too much and exercise too little. Rather, there is a hormonal control mechanism to **utilize, store, or simply waste calories** as the body sees fit. This control mechanism is what matters for weight loss.

Insulin, Glucagon, and the Hypothalamus

The human body has two major hormones which control weight gain and weight loss. These hormones are insulin and glucagon, respectively.

Insulin, a hormone secreted by the pancreas, stimulates fat synthesis and deposition. Simultaneously, it inhibits fat release and oxidation (burning off as energy). Insulin also slows the metabolism. Glucagon, the antagonist hormone to insulin, in contrast, does the exact opposite. It increases the metabolism and stimulates fat breakdown and oxidation, all while inhibiting fat synthesis and deposition.

Both of these hormones act upon the body tissue and hypothalamus to direct a weight "set-point," as well as to direct calories to either be stored as fat or burned as energy. This leads directly to either an increase in adiposity (body fat), or toward a decrease in body fat and a propensity for lean body tissue (thinness). These two hormones, working together with the hypothalamus, direct a sort of "thermostat" for your current weight and body fat level. If you fall below the setting of this thermostat, hunger increases and the body uses every means at its disposal to cause you to gain weight. Similarly, if you exceed this thermostat, the body does all in its power to cause weight loss.

The hormonal obesity theory states that our issue with modern obesity, therefore, is not a result of too many calories and too little exercise, but rather a disruption in the balance of insulin and glucagon. The Yin and Yang, if you will, of Insulin to Glucagon has been disrupted by something we have done in the last 50 years. Prior to 1970, when our obesity epidemic began, these hormones lived in balance, storing fat and burning it in equal measure, directing the hypothalamic weight "thermostat" to keep us at a healthy, normal weight.

Remember the *simplistic* model of obesity states, "Calories eaten that are not burned as energy, cannot otherwise be destroyed, and thus are stored as fat."

The hormonal model of obesity rewrites this in a more sophisticated way, stating, "Calories eaten that are not burned as energy, exhaled as carbon dioxide, urinated out, or utilized for body heat, cannot otherwise be destroyed, and thus are stored as fat. Fat storage, however, is conditional upon the hormonal balance of insulin and glucagon. The decision between caloric wasting and caloric storage is wholly based upon the hormonal state of the body at any given time. Insulin, acting in conjunction with the hypothalamus, induces fat storage and higher body weight, while glucagon, acting in conjunction with the hypothalamus, induces fat loss and lower body weight."

Now that sounds more complete! Put simply, the body can decide whether to store calories as fat or to simply waste them, depending on your hormonal state. Under this theory, we can adequately explain both the traumatic brain injury patient as well as the undiagnosed type 1 diabetic. A traumatic brain injury to the hypothalamus would disrupt weight regulation and the effects of both insulin and glucagon within the body, leading to unrestricted weight gain. Similarly, type 1 diabetes, which is caused by a lack of insulin, results in unmitigated weight loss despite elevated calories ingested. With a more complete model, all of the pieces of the puzzle begin to make sense.

If this hormonal theory of obesity is true, "Eat less, Exercise More" diets are doomed to failure before they begin, as they do not recognize or attempt to affect the hormones which underly the true origin of obesity.

Type 2 Diabetes

If insulin and glucagon direct weight gain and weight loss, what has happened in the last 50 years to affect this so profoundly? The hormonal obesity theory posits that something we have changed in our diet has *increased our insulin levels*, causing weight gain previously unseen in all of human history.

In type 2 diabetes, patients suffer from something called insulin resistance. From a lifestyle of poor eating, their bodies have developed a sort of "tolerance" to insulin. It was the endocrinologist, Dr. Reaven, in his 1988 description of Syndrome X, who first proposed this. As the bodies of type 2 diabetics become more and more "tolerant" or "resistant" to insulin, their body produces *more and more insulin* to counter this resistance. This leads to more hormonal imbalance and more weight gain.

We will discuss insulin, glucagon, and diabetes in more detail later in this book. However, for now, we must try to establish a summary of this theory, which explains our weight gain in the last 50 years. The premise of this book, and indeed the basis of the entire metabolic theory, is this: the foods and food additives which began to take hold since the 1970s, as well as general changes to the way we eat, have led to *ever-increasing insulin levels* in our body. This has led to a never-before-seen imbalance in the hormones of insulin and glucagon. It is for this reason, and this reason alone, that our nation is obese.

The Treatment

Under the hormonal model of obesity, the treatment, therefore, is *not* to eat less and exercise more, but *rather* to target and reduce insulin levels to the ranges which God intended. Our goal is to regain balance and to mimic the hormonal picture of the 1960s human being.

My major purpose in this book is to convince you that our modern diet is designed to do the opposite. The diet of the modern

American is perfectly crafted to cause imbalance. Our modern foods elevate insulin and diminish glucagon, leading to a hormonal state in which all calories are stored as fat, and never wasted. Our imbalance leads us to eat more and more insulin-resistance causing foods throughout our life, effectively keeping us in a weight-gain metabolism day-in, day-out.

By harnessing the natural power of these hormones, and tipping the balance in favor of weight loss, a human being can lose weight effortlessly. And they can do so without calorie restriction or exercise.

I know, it sounds too good to be true. But, trust me, it works! When you begin to lose weight this way, it will seem like magic. I did exactly this and lost 116 pounds. I lost the weight without calorie restriction and without exercise, and so will you.

In the next section, we will evaluate the major changes to the American diet since 1960. As we evaluate each major change, our focus will be on the effect each food has on insulin resistance and hormonal imbalance.

Section II

A Poisoned Food Supply

CHAPTER 4: **FRUCTOSE**

Fructose Overload

How has our food been fundamentally altered since the 1960s, leading to our current obesity epidemic? To begin our investigation of what has changed since the era of effortless weight control, we must first look at one of the biggest changes to the American diet: Sugar. And more specifically, Fructose.

Fructose, as you will see, is present in the American diet at diabolically high levels. What no one talks about, however, is that fructose at high levels within the body has some substantial and dangerous health consequences. During the last 50 years, as America (and the world) has become obese, the amount of fructose in our foods has increased by roughly 1000%. That's right, a tenfold increase! Today, nearly every food you can buy at the grocery store contains "added sugar" or "High Fructose Corn Syrup." Don't believe me? Pick up any product from your pantry which comes in a box or package, and start checking.

Today nearly 95% of our processed or pre-packaged foods contain added sugar, most often in the form of corn syrup. These are often the foods which you would least suspect! Sugar or Corn Syrup can be found, for example, in almost all parts of your sandwich.

There is added sugar in your bread, in your mayonnaise, in your deli meat, and even some cheeses. In your poor little sandwich, only your lettuce and tomato are safe from the food scientists who have added sugar to almost everything.

Chemically, table sugar is indistinguishable from High Fructose Corn Syrup. Both are disaccharides (two-unit sugars) of the same two sugar molecules: glucose and fructose. When your body breaks down table sugar or corn syrup into fructose and glucose, it then has to use each of these smaller units biochemically. Glucose is not a problem. Glucose is familiar to the body.

Fructose, however, is much rarer in nature. It is found almost exclusively in fruit, and in very small amounts. In the body, it is metabolized very similarly to a toxin. Fructose, just like all toxins, can only be metabolized by the liver. Under high doses of fructose, the liver, as the only place where fructose can be metabolized, struggles to keep up with increased metabolic demand.

Throughout the history of humanity, we have always eaten fructose. The difference today is the amount and frequency of our fructose consumption. It far exceeds anything in recorded history!

Pre-world war II, average fructose consumption (mostly from fruit) was between 7-14 grams per day. In the 1970s, after high fructose corn syrup was invented, the average American consumption rose to 37 grams per day. Incidentally, this coincides well with the obesity epidemic, which largely began in 1977.

In 1994 the average American consumption of fructose had risen to 54.7 grams per day. And as of today, Americans eat, on average, nearly 86 grams per day. Do you see a possible connection to our obesity epidemic?

But where did all this increased fructose come from? Why did human beings begin eating fructose in such high concentrations for the first time in human history during the 1970s? Why is there now added sugar or high fructose corn syrup in over 95% of the foods we find on the shelf in the grocery store? In other words, why are

Americans pouring sugar into our mouths like we are giant ants?

We are eating it in our bread, our barbeque sauce, our hamburger buns, our ranch dressing, our mayonnaise, our deli meat, our chips, our taco seasoning packets - you name it! Simply look around, and you will see there is either sugar or high fructose corn syrup in almost everything we package. Even more bizarre, this added sugar is in foods that taste excellent *without* sugar. My own children were stunned when I showed them that their favorite nacho corn chips contained more sugar than salt. (Can you guess the brand?)

This added sugar or high fructose corn syrup accounts for the 1000% increase in our fructose consumption since the 1960s, and a very large aspect of our current obesity crisis.

A Brief History of High Fructose Corn Syrup and the Food Industry

In 1973 Richard Nixon, concerned about his bid for re-election, and the effect which rising food prices would have on his chances at the polls, knew he needed to garner the support of the farming lobby as well as the general public. To accomplish this task, he recruited well-known farm lobbyist Earl Butz to be his Secretary of Agriculture.

Earl "Rusty" Butz was eager to help the president. He began looking for ways to lower food prices, while at the same time, please the farmers. His team had heard of a new product, "high fructose corn syrup," which had been recently invented in 1966 by a scientist at Saga Medical School in Takasaki, Japan. Butz realized, with the invention of corn syrup, he could accomplish both goals simultaneously: increase the value of corn for farmers and lower food prices for the president.

Butz went around tirelessly, speaking with food companies and trying to convince them to substitute normal sugar for high fructose corn syrup in their products. He reasoned with them that the conversion would save them roughly 60% on sugar prices. Eager for better profits, the companies obliged.

Word then spread throughout the food industry that a cheaper substitute for cane sugar existed, and almost overnight, every major company switched from cane sugar to high fructose corn syrup. Since high fructose corn syrup and regular cane sugar are nearly identical chemically, this shouldn't have been a big deal, right? After all, that is what the USDA tells us in its commercials.

That would be true, except that because the high fructose corn syrup was so much cheaper, companies began adding more and more to their products, while keeping their costs the same. The food companies recognized that they could save money even if they doubled or tripled the sugar. This would lead to a tastier product, with a simultaneous cost savings! So why not?

As sugar prices dropped due to their new corn syrup competitor, even the products which did not switch to high fructose corn syrup began to add more sugar. With already rising levels of sugar in our food due to this significantly cheaper sugar alternative, something else happened, which caused an explosion in America's sugar use: the war on fat.

Ancel Keys and the War on Fat

In 1958 Ancel Keys, a Minnesota epidemiologist interested in the cause of heart attacks performed a regression analysis study to try to figure out which foods lead to cardiovascular disease. Ancel Key's "Seven Countries Study" got him on the cover of 1961 Time magazine and has affected nearly 50 years of modern nutrition. The headline finding of his study was this: "Saturated fat leads to heart disease, eat as little saturated fat as possible."

Keys' work led to a cultural shift in America. In the time before the 1970s, butter, lard, beef tallow, duck fat, eggs, and all other animal fats and products were seen as healthy and normal. Almost everyone ate saturated animal fat. However, after the Seven Countries Study, we entered into a culture in which every gram of fat in your diet was seen as toxic. The media and popular culture quickly picked up on a new idea: "Dietary fat makes you fatter and causes heart disease." Before the 1960s, this idea was unheard of.

Many scholars today agree Ancel Keys study was done very poorly. It is well acknowledged that he did not account for other variables of the diets which he studied. The researchers point out that Keys study does not recognize the diets for what they really are: a mix of high-fat, high-sugar.

In the study conclusion, Ancel Keys himself acknowledges that you cannot eliminate the possibility that sugar, not fat, is the actual culprit in the study's findings. Worse still, in an effort to make the data fit the outcome he desired, Ancel Keys deleted several countries from his study results, which showed low rates of heart disease despite high saturated fat intake. His study, initially begun with 22 countries, was pared down to 7 countries for his final results. Contemporary scientists were puzzled. How could a study of Europe exclude France and Germany? These two countries, it should be noted, had very little heart disease at the time despite diets high in saturated fats. It was for this reason Keys deleted them.

Keys numbers were, at best, skewed to show the results he wanted. Regardless of his methods, after his study, Ancel Keys recommended a decrease in dietary fat intake overall, with strict avoidance of saturated fat. Given Keys connections to powerful people on the world stage, including friends at the American Heart Association and American Medical Association, his recommendations quickly became seen as unquestioned scientific fact.

Not everyone agreed, however. At the same time as Ancel Keys, another researcher made a different argument. A man named John Yudkin, diametrically opposed to Ancel Keys, had shown in his research that sugar, and not saturated fat, was to blame for rising heart disease. His book, *Pure, White, and Deadly*, received very little attention compared to the work of Ancel Keys. Yudkin showed how weight gain and heart disease had been accelerating lock-step with the rise of sugar in the modern American diet.

Indeed, in the years from 1700 to 1850, the American diet

included about 5 pounds of sugar per year. As of 1920, this number had increased to 40 lbs. per year. As sugar increased, so did heart disease. Yudkin made the case that saturated fat remained unchanged during this time period, and therefore could not be the culprit. An excellent physiologist and nutritionist, Yudkin showed how excess carbohydrates in the form of sugar are easily converted to triglycerides and fat, leading to obesity and heart disease. Moreover, his own studies into saturated fat showed no correlation between either saturated fat or cholesterol in heart disease.

Because Ancel Keys work had been so readily accepted by a public eager to know the cause of heart disease, Yudkin was ridiculed. The congressional committee responsible for the 1977 Dietary Guidelines was chaired by Senator George McGovern. This committee interviewed Yudkin in 1973, long after most scientific minds in America were made up: fat was bad.

McGovern asked Yudkin if he was truly "suggesting that a high fat intake was not a problem, and that cholesterol presented no danger." In answer to this, Yudkin replied, humbly, "I believe both those things." The committee essentially laughed him out of the hearing, and in 1977, America's dietary recommendations were sealed.

In 1977 the American Heart Association, the American Medical Association, and the United States Department of Agriculture all came out in one voice, recommending we lower our total dietary fat consumption from 40% to 30% and avoid saturated animal fats. The case was closed, and the matter settled: our wise politicians had sided with Ancel Keys, and fat, not sugar, was to blame for our heart disease.

But for the processed food industry, Ancel Keys recommendations became like handcuffs. Overnight, Americans, afraid of heart disease and stroke (and rightly so), tried to listen to their supposed wise medical community and reduce or eliminate fat from their diets. The United States went crazy for "Low-Fat." There was a sudden demand from the public for food companies to produce fat-free and low-fat versions of all foods. Fat-free dressing, low-fat mayonnaise, fat-free cookies, and every other conceivable food that could be made in a fat-free form was suddenly in high demand. Food companies began to print "fat-free" on every box label they created, even if the food never had fat to begin with.

We entered a bizarre era in which people would say ridiculous things like: "Gummy bears are good for you; they are fat-free!". Labels on factory-made food would boast "Naturally fat-free" as if there is anything natural about a processed candy! This cultural shift led to "healthy cookies" packaged in "healthy green wrappers," low in fat but high in sugar, and a host of other crazy "low-fat" foods which lined the grocery store shelves starting in the early 1980s.

But what happens to processed food, made in an American factory, when you take all the fat out? Well, to be blunt, it tastes like crap! And American food companies knew this. To rectify the situation, they added the one thing no-one was talking about that helped to improve the taste of disgusting, fatless, processed foods: they added sugar. And more specifically, they added high fructose corn syrup.

One of my favorite examples is the "Baked Chip" (I bet you can guess the brand). This product, made by squeezing out a sugary paste into "chip" form, is so naturally bland and disgusting due to the deletion of fats from its ingredient list, that its producer has added sugar to levels which boggle the mind. Indeed, to cover up the amount of sugar in each serving size, the producers have labeled sugar in four different ways, just to try to disguise it a little bit! Instead of listing sugar as the main ingredient, it lists Dextrose, Sugar, Corn Syrup, and Maltodextrin. All are types of sugar.

Whether Ancel Key's fudged his study or not, one thing is clear: since Ancel Keys made his recommendations, obesity and heart disease have sky-rocketed. Let's ask ourselves: Was the American Heart Association right? Was the American Medical Association right? Are we better off than we were in 1960? In 1977, they recommended we drop our dietary fat to 30%, and we did. In fact, we surpassed that, and by some studies, we dropped to less than 25% of our calories from fat. Meanwhile, our carbohydrate consumption increased. Looking around at our world, do you think Ancel Keys, or his contemporary ideological enemy, John Yudkin, was actually correct? Personally, I side with Yudkin!

Years after Ancel Keys Seven Countries study, an Italian researcher named Alessandro Menotti went back to the data and found that the food in the study which most correlated with deaths from heart disease was not fat, but rather sugar. Think about that for a moment. If the study actually showed sugar, and in particular fructose, was to blame for our worsening heart disease, what had the major organizations just done by eliminating fat and replacing it with sugar? They had essentially just doubled and tripled down on the problem. Is that compatible with the problems we see around us today?

Since these recommendations came out, what grade should we give the associations who recommended them? How is our heart disease going? Our diabetes? Our High Blood Pressure? Stroke? The prevalence of all of these diseases is through the roof! All markers of metabolic syndrome have gotten worse. We are sicker, fatter, and our cardiovascular health is far worse with an increase in sugar and a decrease in dietary fat. Yet still, the medical community is slow to address the possibility that sugar, and specifically fructose, may be toxic.

Your Body on Fructose

In your body's metabolism, fructose can only be metabolized by the liver and in a very special way: essentially in the same way as alcohol. Alcohol in the body is converted readily to a metabolite called acetyl-CoA, which then overloads a biochemical pathway in the liver to create triglycerides (fats). These triglycerides are then either stored in the liver, stored on your body as adipose (fatty) tissue, or directed toward your bloodstream where they circulate as elevated triglyceride levels.

Have you ever seen a beer belly? Have you ever wondered why it exists? A beer belly exists because alcohol is essentially only processed into fat, which your body then stores. If there is a beer belly from alcohol, and alcohol is processed in the same way as fructose, it stands to reason there is such a thing as a fructose belly.

Studies have shown that glucose causes almost no denovo lipogenesis (your body creating new fat). The same calories given as fructose, on the other hand, can double the amount of new fat created by your body.

In one of my favorite studies, completed in 2005, participants were instructed to consume 25% of their calories as fructose, while the control group consumed 25% of their calories as glucose. The study ran for 10 weeks. Within 2 months of beginning their new dietary instructions, both groups had gained weight. However, there was a substantial difference in the amount! The glucose group had gained only 3 lbs. The fructose group, meanwhile, had gained 17 lbs and had developed non-alcoholic fatty liver. Non-alcoholic fatty liver is a disease in which your liver embeds fat throughout the entirety of the liver tissue, leading to liver dysfunction.

Furthermore, the fructose group experienced decreased fat metabolism, decreased metabolic rate, increased uric acid (gout), increased insulin resistance, increased triglycerides, increased LDL cholesterol, and increased blood tests which signify liver strain. Essentially, the fructose group began to experience the typical symptom profile of a person with metabolic syndrome, formerly "Syndrome X"! This cannot be overstated!

Are you beginning to see the picture? If we are eating a substance at rates 1000% higher than our predecessors in 1950 and 1960, and this substance converts almost entirely to triglycerides and LDL cholesterol, what affect might this have on our body weight and cholesterol levels? What about our heart disease?

In medical school, Non-Alcoholic Fatty Liver is taught as something called "NASH" syndrome or Non-Alcoholic Steato-Hepatitis. For a long time, NASH syndrome has perplexed physicians. Medical students are taught that the origin of NASH syndrome is not fully known. In alcohol-related liver disease, the mechanism of disease is thought to be very well understood. NASH, however, remains a mystery. But what if the answer is simply fructose? What if a metabolite processed similarly to alcohol, which exists in almost all of our foods, can lead to a liver dysfunction similar to alcoholism? Today roughly 20% of Americans have some degree of non-alcoholic fatty liver disease. Does this fit with our increased fructose consumption?

In the above study, the fructose consuming group, after returning to their normal diet, saw a return to normal healthy livers and a correction of all metabolic dysfunction. Do you still want to eat this stuff? Because it is in *everything*!

Fructose Causes Many Problems

Further studies have shown fructose is 7 times more likely to form AGED's. AGED's stand for Advanced Glycation End Products. This name seems complicated, but in actuality, it is simple. When your blood glucose levels run high, glucose can "stick" to things. A linkage referred to as an AGED is a chemical cross-link between glucose and a protein in the body. Glucose can stick to almost any protein, whether they be in your retina, your kidney, your blood vessels, or even your red blood cells.

No doubt, you have heard that diabetes can lead to blindness, kidney failure, amputation, nerve damage, and a host of the other problems associated with poor blood glucose control. These AGEDs are the cause. And fructose increases their rate by 700%!

Further studies have shown fructose does not inhibit ghrelin release. Ghrelin, a hormone secreted by your stomach, is a potent hunger signal within the body. Fat, protein, and even glucose tell your stomach to turn this hunger signal off. Fructose does not. And it is in 95% of our food!

Fructose has also been shown to inhibit leptin. Leptin, as we will discuss later, is the most potent hunger suppressant in the body. It tells the brain to shut-down any hunger drive, and has even been shown to switch our body into "fat-burning mode." Fructose inhibits its action.

But most importantly for our study on obesity, Fructose has been linked to insulin resistance. As we will discuss later, Insulin is vitally important to your weight. When your body is resistant to its natural insulin, your pancreas secretes higher and higher amounts in an attempt to obtain the same hormonal result. As insulin promotes fat storage, this leads to ever-increasing levels of obesity.

Because of the above findings, it should be of no surprise that fructose consumption in study after study has led to obesity. In a 2010 study evaluating fructose consumption in rats, scientists compared rats fed sucrose (50% fructose) vs. pure fructose (100% fructose). In the fructose-fed rats, the rats became obese within 8 weeks, gaining significantly more weight than the sucrose rats. The rats also developed severe insulin resistance after only 2 weeks on the high fructose diet.

This study is of particular concern, as food companies have recently begun to use something called "Crystalline Fructose" in American food. Both sugar and corn syrup are roughly 50% fructose. Crystalline Fructose, however, is 100% pure fructose. This new sweetener, unseen in human history, is currently being added to American foods in an effort to increase sweetness and subsequently enhance the hunger drive of consumers. With the addition of crystalline fructose, our American diet has leaned even further into insanity.

Added Sugar in Your Food

Your homework is to look around the grocery store at ingredients and try to spot added sugar. Many foods contain natural sugar, such as tomatoes. But that is not our concern. I want you to look for sugar added unnecessarily. This will be listed, under current FDA guidelines, separately from the main ingredient. For example, the main ingredient of spaghetti sauce should be tomatoes, followed by spices and seasonings. Below is a commonly sold American Spaghetti Sauce.

As you can see from the nutritional facts, the product contains sugar. In general, this is okay. Unless specifically stated, this may simply be the natural sugar from the tomatoes. To see if any sugar has been added unnecessarily by the food companies, we must look at the ingredient list. Which, for this product, looks like this:

Nutrition Facts

Serv. Size 1/2 Cup (125g)
Servings about 5

Amount Per Serving

Calories 80	Fat Cal. 35

	% Daily Value*
Total Fat 4g	**6%**
Sat. Fat 0.5g	**3%**
Trans Fat 0g	
Cholest. 0mg	**0%**
Sodium 420mg	**18%**
Total Carb. 8g	**3%**
Dietary Fiber 2g	**10%**
Sugars 5g	
Protein 2g	

Vitamin A 20%	•	Vitamin C 30%
Calcium 6%	•	Iron 15%

* Percent Daily Values (DV) are based on a 2,000 calorie diet.

Ingredients: Tomato Puree (Water, Tomato Paste), Soybean Oil, Salt, **Sugar**, Dehydrated Onions, Extra Virgin Olive Oil, Spices, Natural Flavors.

The ingredient list indicates that the manufacturer has added extra sugar, beyond that found in tomatoes, as the fourth highest ingredient in this product. **This is not okay**. There is no need for this extra sugar.

The first goal of this book is to recognize and eliminate foods which add sugar to their products. We simply do not want the harmful effects which unnecessarily added fructose produces. Why would we put a stumbling block of extra fructose in front of our effort to lose weight, and reclaim our insulin sensitivity? But to this end, we must be wise.

The food companies purposely divide sugar into several different names. Why do they do this? Simply put, they do not want to list sugar as the main ingredient. Under FDA guidelines, the highest prevalence ingredient in a food must be listed first. By splitting the added sugar into four different "types of sugar," the food companies can list these four ingredients as 5th, 6th, 7th, and 8th, rather than just smacking "Sugar" down as ingredient number 1. They think we are too stupid to recognize this.

Added Sugar is given many names in ingredient lists today. The majority of them are listed below:

Sugar, Cane Sugar, Evaporated Cane Juice, Fruit Juice, Fruit Juice Concentrate, Castor Sugar, Coconut Sugar, Confectioners or Powdered Sugar, Corn Syrup, High Fructose Corn Syrup, Corn Syrup Solids, Crystalline Fructose, Date Sugar, Demerara Sugar, Dextrin, Dextrose, Fructose, Galactose, Maltose, Sucrose, Beet Sugar, Brown Sugar, Cane Juice Crystals, Florida Crystals, Golden Sugar, Glucose Syrup Solids, Grape Sugar, Icing Sugar, Maltodextrin, Muscovado Sugar, Panela Sugar, Raw Sugar, Granulated Sugar, Table Sugar, Turbinado Sugar, Yellow Sugar, Agave Nectar, Agave Syrup, Barley Malt, Blackstrap Molasses, Brown Rice Syrup, Buttered Sugar/Buttercream, Caramel, Carob Syrup, Golden Syrup, Honey, Invert Sugar, Maple Syrup, Molasses, Rice Syrup, Refiner's Syrup, Sorghum Syrup

And they are figuring out more names for the stuff every day. My favorite is "Free Trade Cane Sugar." I suppose if they are trying to poison you, they might as well add the words "Free Trade" to make you feel like a humanitarian.

If sugar is listed separately, it is then considered "added" sugar. For the most part, the things to which God added sugar are perfectly fine for you. Take an orange, for example. It has 15 g of sugar, 3 g of which is fructose. However, unlike modern processed food, it is packaged (as we will discuss later) with fiber. This fiber nullifies the harmful burst of fructose to the system. God, you will find, is pretty smart. Humans are dumb. We ruin our food before eating it. God knows about anything that may harm you, and so he packages it exactly as your body needs it. Fructose, studies have shown, causes no problems at low levels. But the levels at which we eat it today are above all levels seen in human history. Today we eat 17% of our calories from fructose. To achieve this same amount from fruit, you would have to eat 27 oranges every day!

When you look at the ingredient list of your foods, try to avoid those which list any of the above types of sugar. Sugar which is listed in the ingredients as a separate addition of the manufacturer is purely designed to increase taste at the expense of your health.

This leads us to rule #1 of Dr. Cimino's Weight Loss Solution:

Rule #1: I will not eat any product with *added* sugar, nor will I eat any product with High Fructose Corn Syrup.

Next, we will look at another enormous change to the American diet, which occurred almost simultaneously with our switch to high-sugar consumption. Let's look at the disaster of Omega-6 Vegetable Oils.

CHAPTER 5: **SOPPING IN VEGETABLE OIL**

Our Fats Changed!

Since the dawn of recorded history, human beings have had only two options for the fats used in cooking. Firstly, and most prominently, human beings could obtain their fats from animals. This came either in the form of fat from the animal meat itself or in the form of butter.

Secondly, humans could obtain oil from certain plant foods which were naturally oily, or laden with fat. Because humans had no factories in which to perform complicated procedures to extract fat, only the oiliest and most easily "pressed" plant sources could be used.

Olives, for example, express natural olive oil when squeezed within a fruit press. Coconuts are filled with a solid white fatty substance which can be scraped out and used for cooking. Animal fats are readily removed from meat. This fat melts easily in a pan, adds tremendous flavor, and enhances almost all cooked and baked goods. Butter needs no explanation! These fats, my friends, are the ones your body was made to eat.

Access to fats has always been necessary for cooking. But because only certain places on earth had access to coconuts, palms, or olives, the vast majority of humanity throughout time relied almost exclusively on animal fat to get the job done.

Simply put, for all of human history, there was no other source of dietary fat which could be used for cooking. That is, of course, until the 20th century. Throughout the 20th century, our dietary fat source began to mutate. Once natural and obvious, the science of which fats were ok and which fats were harmful became obscured and confused. People were told, for the first time in recorded memory, to avoid "saturated fats," and offered in their place synthetic oils, created in a factory.

As you will see, in the age before rampant American obesity, the average American didn't buy products soaked with "vegetable oil." They didn't use baking sprays made entirely of soybean oil. If they wanted butter, they got a stick from the fridge and spread it on their toast, by gosh! So, what changed? To look at how the fats in our diet were fundamentally altered, we have to start in the 1800s.

A Brief History of Seed Oils

In the 1800s, we began to need oil. America and the world had just gone through an industrial revolution which brought us some amazing new machines: steam engines and factory lines, trains, cotton gins, steamboats, and all kinds of iron behemoths. And as you well know, these items require something to keep them running smoothly. They require oil.

From the 1820s through the 1860s, we primarily obtained this oil from whaling. Whales were hunted down, and their oil was processed and shipped out as machine oil. But there are only so many whales! The whale population quickly began to deteriorate, and we soon found there were not enough whales left to support our ever-burgeoning industrial society. So, we did what humans do best: we found a different resource.

In 1857, at the height of the American cotton industry, the cotton producers had an "Aha!" moment. They realized they had missed a potential revenue source for years, right under their noses. A byproduct of their cotton production was oil!

In 1857 William Fee invented an automatic huller, which efficiently separated the tough hulls from the cottonseeds. The cottonseeds could then be used for oil extraction. Before this automatic huller, the process of creating oil from cottonseeds was arduous and time-consuming, and the profit was not worth the effort. After this invention, however, cottonseed oil began to be used as a supplement for diminishing whale oil. It was used to light street lamps, for lubrication, and for soap.

In 1911, food scientists were successful in stabilizing (turning solid) the oil produced by the cottonseed. This chemical process created a white fatty substance which looked both like soap and a bit like lard. The scientists discussed what they might do with the substance. Could they sell it as soap? They considered the possibility, but this was already being done, and the profits weren't great. Suddenly they had an idea. They decided to create a new "synthetic lard" made of cottonseed oil to replace natural pig lard. They would market it as safer, better, and cleaner than conventional pig fat.

The subsequent campaign to replace natural pig-lard was extremely successful. Entire cookbooks were sold with all animal fats replaced by synthetic lard. This new seed oil-based "lard" swept the nation like a fever. It built further steam after Upton Sinclair's famous book, *The Jungle*. In *The Jungle*, Sinclair shed light on the food industry's often cruel treatment of animals. For the food scientists of the age, this was the perfect opportunity to replace "evil lard and tallow," with humane, scientific, and futuristic laboratory fats. And it worked!

Almost overnight, millennia of eating beef tallow, pig lard, and churned animal butter began to be replaced by a non-food seed oil, chemically altered to be stable. Over the next 30 years up to 1940, companies would begin to use other seeds, and other oils, but the process was the same: a seed would be placed under tremendous pressure and heat to extract oil which God never meant for us to eat.

In 1940, it was discovered how to create seed oils which are stable enough for the grocery shelf. Previously cottonseed oil had been too temperamental to sell on a mass scale; it quickly went rancid and could not survive long-term shipping and storage. But, with new chemical techniques, this problem could be circumvented. Rather than a white lardy substance, companies were now able to create a synthetic golden-colored oil marketable to the American public. This allowed the food companies to sell the oils we see today: Canola, Soybean, Safflower, Grapeseed, Corn, and so on.

Later, these oils were purposefully rebranded as "vegetable oils" to obscure their true source: Seeds. Think about all of the oils you see in products today: Safflower Seed Oil, Sunflower Seed Oil, Canola (seed) oil, Soybean Oil. Did you hear any "vegetable" names? If you are like me, you had to research to learn what the heck a "Canola" is anyway!

Despite increasing popularity, the use of these oils was still quite limited throughout the early 1900s and remained a minor factor in the American diet until the 1970s. During the 1970s, the ingestion of these oils became a revolution in human dietary history.

The War on Saturated Fat

In 1961 and again in 1971, following the work of Ancel Keys, the American Heart Association made its recommendation that Americans replace saturated animal fat with polyunsaturated vegetable oils. After the recommendations of the American Heart Association, the housewife of the late 1960s and early 1970s began to replace butter and lard with margarine (made entirely of seed oils). Saturated animal fats were demonized country-wide, and a subsequent campaign was waged to get saturated fats out of things like popcorn at the movie theater, fast food fryers, and cooking tops at restaurants. Almost overnight, instead of getting movie popcorn with real butter, or a restaurant steak seared in lard, you got a heaping helping of vegetable oil.

Until the 1990s, even McDonald's fried its fries in beef tallow rather than in "vegetable oil." Everyone who has tasted beef-tallow French fries states they were, frankly, exceptional. Many wish they would return to this recipe! But even McDonald's could not withstand the societal pressure of nutritional "experts" who insisted we abandon the saturated fat we had eaten for millennia.

Sadly, there was no data then to support this transition, and there remains no data today. On the contrary, there have been hundreds of well-organized, randomized controlled studies which have shown that replacing saturated fats with poly-unsaturated vegetable oil does not improve cardiovascular mortality.

Moreover, there have been numerous studies which have linked diets rich in poly-unsaturated vegetable oils with higher incidences of inflammation, cancer, gallstones, stroke, and cirrhosis of the liver.

After Ancel keys made his recommendation, several well-funded studies were enacted to study the effects of men on diets in which saturated fats had been replaced with poly-unsaturated fats. These studies included the NIH Funded Multiple Risk Factor Intervention (MRFIT) Trial, the L.A. Veterans Trial, and the Oslo Diet Heart study.

Of these three studies, all showed that reducing saturated fat reduced cholesterol. But what about mortality? On the issue of death, the studies were far less impressive. The MRFIT trial, for example, found no statistically significant difference in mortality between a group eating primarily poly-unsaturated vegetable oil, and those eating the normal saturated animal fats.

Worse yet, the men who replaced their dietary fat entirely with vegetable oils had slightly lower cholesterol but had almost triple the rate of cancer, an increase in weight, gallstones, liver issues and a host of other problems. Even more alarming, in the Sydney Diet Heart Study, the substitution of saturated fat with vegetable oil *increased* the rates of cardiac death.

This was so concerning to the National Health Institute that meetings were called with the researchers of the day to discuss these troubling findings. They reviewed these concerning results at length, made excuses, but ultimately decided "we must be right," despite the data. They went on to fully endorse polyunsaturated vegetable oils for heart health, with a goal of lowering total cholesterol.

How Much Vegetable Oil Are We Eating?

Vegetable oils are anything but natural. They are extracted under tremendous heat, after which they turn a greyish-white color and become foul-smelling. Vegetable oils are then chemically treated to deodorize the putrid smell, further chemically treated for clarity, and finally dyed a false golden color. When they ship to the grocery store, they look almost like something edible. But these oils were unknown to humanity for all of the millennia up until the 1900s. Today they appear in almost all processed foods.

Over the decades since 1960, obesity and the use of synthetic "Vegetable Oils" have risen in tandem. Though we cannot say definitively that two matching charts equal causality, it is hard to ignore the correlation.

Here is a graph of humanity's increase in vegetable oils, overlaid with our rise in obesity. Also, notice the decline in butter use:

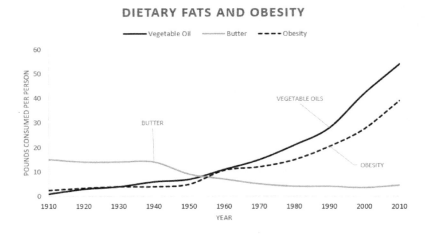

Today, 76% of American foods on the store shelves contain vegetable oil, as well as nearly 100% of fast-food restaurants. Almost all sit-down restaurant chains fry their meat in vegetable oil. Due to the many sources and expansive use of this unnatural fat, vegetable oil consumption by modern Americans has increased 1,400% since 1960. Yes, you read that correctly. Fourteen Hundred Percent increase in vegetable oil consumption since 1960!

Over the same time period, as we have already shown, obesity has increased by 400%. Is there a possible connection?

It is hard to ignore the rise in obesity and the rise in vegetable oil, which happened almost simultaneously. The question becomes: what do these synthetically created oils, which were unknown to human metabolism before 1900, do to our body? Do studies support the possibility that vegetable oils lead to obesity and insulin resistance?

Your Body on Seed Oil

In a 2015 study, mice were separated into different feeding groups. Each group was given the exact same number of calories; however, one group was fed a diet composed primarily of vegetable oil, while another group was fed a diet rich in saturated fat. A third control group was fed "standard mice chow." Their weight, insulin resistance, inflammatory markers, and liver health were all compared over 32 weeks.

The results were astounding. The mice eating vegetable oils became obese, ***doubling*** the weights of their counterparts eating ***the same number of calories*** as saturated fat. This led the researchers to conclude that vegetable oils are an "Obesogen." An obesogen is a substance that directly causes obesity. In this particular study, the vegetable oil was Soybean. Today, soybean oil is the most prevalent vegetable oil in the modern American diet.

Worse yet, the mice fed vegetable oil showed considerably higher levels of insulin resistance. As the hormonal imbalance of insulin is the major driver of obesity in our time, this has significant relevance to the modern American.

Vegetable oil also has a profound impact on inflammation. A 2013 study showed that mice fed foods high in polyunsaturated vegetable oil had elevated weight gain, increased appetite, and higher fatty tissue inflammation. Inflammation has been shown in study after study to lead directly to insulin resistance, which further leads to obesity.

Omega 6 vs. Omega 3

As more data comes out on vegetable oils, their effects become more and more alarming. But not all poly-unsaturated fats are bad. Vegetable oils are not the only way that our bodies obtain poly-unsaturated fatty acids. In fact, these fats are essential to life, and part of a healthy wholesome diet.

In the normal human diet, poly-unsaturated fats are found in all plant matter as well as in all animal meat. They only become toxic in their industrial conversion to huge bottles of mass-produced oil, bought in bulk from the store shelves, or cooked into our processed foods in amazingly high quantities. Like fructose, God put these oils naturally in the human diet. Humanity, as usual, took a good thing, bastardized it, and turned it into something harmful.

In medicine, we further delineate the type of poly-unsaturated oils into two groups. These are known as Omega 3 and Omega 6 fatty acids.

In nature, Omega 3 fatty acids are found in higher frequency in marine life, grass, seaweed, algae, and green leaves. Today many people take algae, flaxseed, or fish oil supplements to try to increase their Omega 3 fatty acids, as these fats predominate in the human brain. They are thought to increase cognitive function, as well as to help stave off dementia.

Omega 6 fatty acids, conversely, are found in seeds and grains. They naturally occur in wheat, barley, soybeans, corn, and all of the substances from which we gather oils today. Importantly, no mass-produced oil in the American diet is rich in Omega 3. All oils currently used in processed food are rich in Omega 6.

While Omega 3 fatty acid has been linked to the reduction of inflammation, as well as many protective effects for the brain, Omega 6 fatty acid has been extensively linked to whole-body inflammation. These two fats fight each other. One promotes inflammation, and the other reduces it. What matters is the ratio between the two.

In the preindustrial era, the Omega 6 to Omega 3 ratio in the American diet was around 2:1. This nearly-equal ratio balanced out the body's inflammation. In 1960 it had climbed to 3:1. However, today, after the world-wide spread of vegetable oils and the 1,400% rise in their consumption, the ratio of Omega 6 to Omega 3 in the American diet is estimated at 76:1! If Omega 6 causes inflammation, and Omega 3 cures inflammation, what might a 76:1 ratio be doing to our bodies? This ratio has never been seen in human history!

The Omega 6 to Omega 3 ratio of the modern American is so high that anyone taking Omega 3 supplements from fish oil might as well be "pissing in the wind." You will never overcome a 76:1 ratio by supplementing Omega 3. The only hope you have is to drastically reduce your Omega 6 intake. And you do that by getting rid of vegetable oils.

The Fats of Today

Below is a graph of the commonly used fats in modern America, and their respective ratio of Omega-6. For the purposes of my diet, I specifically tried to eliminate dietary fats high in Omega 6. After implementing the dietary changes within this book, I reduced my insulin needs by 95% over three months, and over six months lost 116 lbs. This move away from Omega 6-rich vegetable oils, in my opinion, was a huge part of this success.

OMEGA-6 CONTENT OF FATS

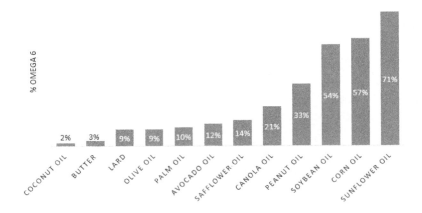

As you see, all fats contain some component of Omega 6, but some have considerably higher amounts. It is these which we must avoid.

Omega 9

You have already read the effects of Omega 6 and Omega 3 fatty acids, but what is an Omega 9? You may know Omega 9 by its most famous name: Olive Oil. Omega 9, or oleic acid, is known as a mono-unsaturated fat. Neither fully a saturated fat (solid at room temperature) nor fully poly-unsaturated (such as vegetable oil), the oleic acid contains one single unsaturated bond in its chemical structure.

Olive oil, the most prominent mono-unsaturated fat (Omega 9 Oleic Acid) has been studied extensively. In almost all research, it has been shown to benefit the body in amazing ways. It has been linked to reduced rates of cancer, increased arterial elasticity, and protection from heart disease and stroke. But even more impressive for our purpose of weight loss, olive oil has been linked to a reduction in insulin resistance!

Because Omega 9 fatty acid (olive oil) and saturated fat (animal fat) do not factor into the inflammatory struggle between Omega 6 and Omega 3, their consumption does not lead to detrimental effects.

By contrast, soybean oil is almost entirely Omega-6 fatty acid. It also happens to be the most heavily used oil in the American diet.

You are What You Eat

In a very interesting study spanning the decades from 1961 to 2008, fat samples taken from humans over each decade were compared against each other. The researchers were able to compare the content of the subject's body fat, and the results are startling.

In 1961, the percentage of our body fat made up of Omega 6 fatty acids comprised less than 8% of total body fat. In 2008, it comprised over 25% No one knows what it is today, or will be in 2025.

But humans are not the only ones who have succumb to this change. In the 1950s and 1960s, it was much more common to eat grass-fed beef. Throughout the 1970s and 1980s, corn-fed, rather than grass-fed beef, began to gain popularity. If Omega 3 fatty acids come from grass, and corn gives predominantly Omega 6 fatty acids, might another source of our dietary Omega 6 be our meat? Indeed, it is!

In a major study done on the fatty acid content of modern beef, researchers found a predominance of Omega 6 fatty acids. In corn-fed beef, the Omega 6 to Omega 3 ratio was found to be roughly 9:1. Grass-fed beef, in contrast, has a ratio of roughly 2:1.

We see this trend in grain-fed chicken and eggs as well. As chicken and beef are the two predominant types of meat in modern America, it is becoming increasingly difficult to avoid high levels of Omega 6 fatty acids.

Thankfully, there is a modern movement to return to pasture-raised chicken and eggs, as well as grass-fed beef. Of this movement, I am a full subscriber. I advise you to become one as well!

Our Rule

To undo the damage done by the dietary changes since the 1960s, we must certainly take into account this dramatic shift in the dietary fats of the modern American. For this reason, we must pause here and define our next rule for maximal weight loss.

Rule # 2: I will not eat "Vegetable Oils" rich in Omega 6 fatty acids. When I need oil for cooking, I will use Olive Oil or Avocado Oil. When I cook with heat, I will simply use butter.

As you look at packaged food in our modern era, you will notice that most processed food contains a vegetable oil derived from seeds. Scan the ingredient list for Soybean Oil, Safflower Seed Oil, Sunflower Seed Oil, Peanut Oil, and Corn Oil. If any of these is listed, simply move on. Rules 1 and 2 alone will have a dramatic effect on your weight. But to truly heal our insulin resistance, we must push further.

Important Point:

Today many olive oils have been corrupted with the addition of soybean oils. Do not use "Light" olive oil or any product which simply says "olive oil." Instead, use only Extra Virgin Olive Oil.

It is also best to use "Cold Pressed Oils." Cold Pressed means the oil is extracted without the addition of heat. Heat is used to get every extra drop of oil out of an olive or another oil-producing plant. When this occurs, many of the beneficial substances present in olives are destroyed by the heat. These substances are known as phenols and are very delicate. But their health benefits are amazing. It is possible these substances are responsible for olive oil's amazing benefits on arteries, cancer reduction, and insulin resistance.

CHAPTER 6: **REFINED CARBOHYDRATES AND FIBER**

The Fullness Dilemma

I want you to perform a mental exercise. I am going to offer you three foods, and we will compare the impulses of your body. First, I'd like to offer you a meal of a half cup of olive oil. We will add some salt for flavor. Interested? Or does the idea slightly nauseate you?

If you said nauseated, you answered similarly to almost all human beings on this planet, and likely any human being in our history. The body is very good at regulating fat intake. After eating high fat, your body will signal you with a hormone called Cholecystokinin, which acts potently in the brain to tell you have had enough food. Likewise, fats do not cause neurotransmitters to signal "cravings." Thus, you can confidently walk away from an offer of pure oil.

Second, let me offer you one pound of cooked ground turkey — no sauce, or sides, or vegetables. Just one pound of ground turkey browned in a frying pan. Do you feel like snacking on this for an hour or so? Likely not. Similar to fat, the body has excellent brain mechanisms for telling you that you are full, or not interested to begin with, in high amounts of protein. After eating protein, your body will release a hormone called Peptide YY, which turns hunger almost completely off. Likewise, if the body does not need calories or nutrients from meat, the brain effectively turns off your interest in such foods. So far, so good.

Now let me offer you a third food. Picture your favorite carbohydrate. Perhaps it is potato chips? Popcorn? French Fries? Maybe it is a bagel. Or how about a chewy French baguette? Maybe, like me, you enjoy pretzels. I am willing to bet you already feel the tug of hunger as you picture your favorite carbohydrate. Most human beings find that when they feel hungry, or desire to snack, it is almost always carbohydrates which draw their longing. Likewise, once eating, it is almost always carbohydrates which cause the most problems when trying to *stop* eating.

Let's do another mental scenario. Picture yourself at a restaurant, out to dinner with your extended family. You have just finished your meal, and you feel decently full. The conversation lags onward as you wait for your family to finish eating. At the center of the table, there is a basket full of bread. Could you possibly eat some more bread to help pass the time? Studies have shown you can.

In multiple studies, human subjects declined further portions of fats and protein when full, but almost always had room for further carbohydrates. No one ever has the urge to drink a tablespoon of oil while waiting for their companions to finish their meals, but put some bread on the table, and they will snack for hours.

In fact, this has even earned the term "the second stomach effect." The second stomach effect is defined as the propensity for a human being to suddenly find room for dessert, after being completely satisfied and filled by their dinner. The phrase "there is always room for Jell-O" is true! Human beings, stuffed to the gills, can find room for carbohydrates when the dessert bell is rung. So, what gives? Did God forget to give the human body a mechanism to turn off carbohydrate hunger, but yet designed fat and protein perfectly? As I have said often, God is pretty smart. Is it likely he forgot carbohydrates? Or more likely we have somehow ruined them, much in the same way we have ruined fats?

The trick to understanding why we seem to have no mechanism to turn off carbohydrate hunger is to understand the missing ingredient. God doesn't forget anything, and he didn't forget about carbohydrates. The system is, in a word, perfect. Carbohydrates are no exception. We simply took out a key ingredient. We took out fiber.

To prove the point, let me offer you a fourth snack. Let's try some carbohydrates with fiber. I'd like to offer you three full stalks of broccoli. I'll even cook it in butter and salt. Interested? Or do you feel slightly repulsed as you did with the half cup of olive oil or the one pound of ground turkey? Ok, I'll make the offer better. How about 4 sweet potatoes, cooked with butter and salt? Still not interested? How about 3 bowls of oatmeal? Would that sound like a good snack? While I'm certain your salivary glands are yawning at the prospect of broccoli or oatmeal, a human can eat a full bag of barbeque potato chips without blinking. And many Americans do just that at lunch time.

Once Upon a Time, All Carbohydrates Had Fiber

Once upon a time, all carbohydrates in the human diet had fiber. It is estimated that in the paleolithic period of humanity when we operated as hunter-gatherers, humans ate roughly 100 g of dietary fiber per day. That is a lot of fiber! Today the modern American eats a pitiful 15 grams per day. Though our modern intake of fiber is pathetic, this change makes perfect sense.

If the only carbohydrates available to ancient man came in the form of natural wild fruits and vegetables, the fiber content in the ancient diet would have been tremendous. As humanity operated primarily as hunter-gatherers, the diet consisted mostly of meats, saturated animal fats, and scavenged berries, nuts, and root vegetables. Because these are all-natural whole foods, without any processing done in a factory, their fiber content is perfect for maintaining optimal digestion, insulin sensitivity, and fullness.

After the paleolithic era of the hunter-gatherer, humanity figured out how to operate agrarian societies. We moved from hunting and gathering to domesticating animals for husbandry, and planting our preferred fruits, vegetables, and grains for later harvesting. Over the last 6,000 years, grain has become a principal part of the human diet.

Throughout history, no matter where on the Earth a human has lived, there has been a primary grain. In Asia and Sub-Asia, the primary grain has been rice. In North and South America, the ancient historical grain was corn. In Europe, humans relied primarily on wheat, barley, and oats. All of these products can be eaten in their whole form or can be processed into something much more refined.

During refinement, the whole grain, no matter which, is milled into a powder which can then be used to bake alternate products. Corn, for example, can be milled into corn flour which is then used to make corn bread or tortillas. Today, in modern America, our preferred refined carbohydrate of choice is wheat.

Wheat flour is created by milling wheat berries. Wheat berries are the natural edible portion of the wheat plant. A wheat berry consists of a wheat millet, a wheat head, and a wheat germ. Within these portions of the wheat berry are natural fats, proteins, and, of course, fiber. In ancient times, flour was hand-milled using stone tools. When milled, the natural flour preserved these portions of the grain. This led to bread and wheat-products which were high in fiber, extremely filling, and minimally detrimental to insulin resistance.

In the 1870s, during the period of the industrial revolution, ancient milling techniques were replaced with industrial factory milling. In this new milling process, companies were suddenly able to isolate and extract the wheat head from the wheat berry, separating off the wheat germ, the wheat bran, and the wheat millet. What had started out as a whole food, designed to protect you from all the detriments of dietary imbalance, instantly became a food which is very close to pure sugar!

As the production of flour advanced, food companies became even better at removing all of the bran from the flour. They then began bleaching the flour with a chlorine formula to get the attractive white powder which we all consider classic, normal flour today. This new white powder more closely resembled cocaine than classic wheat flour!

As this new product contained almost no fiber, nor any protein or natural fats, its ability to increase glucose levels in the bloodstream became very potent. Rather than having its glucose absorption slowed by competing fiber, protein, and fat, refined white flour breaks down quickly into subunits of glucose. This begins in the saliva of the mouth and continues throughout the stomach and intestines. The units of glucose then cause massive spikes in blood glucose levels. Subsequently, these glucose spikes cause huge spikes in insulin levels, which then stimulate body-fat creation, body-fat preservation, and, of course, insulin resistance! Even worse, this refined flour creates almost no sensation of fullness.

At the Cimino home, we performed an experiment. We obtained whole wheat berries and did our best to hand-mill them into enough flour to bake one loaf of bread. The results astounded us. The loaf of bread was extraordinarily dense and grainy tasting. After about two bites, we were full! It was the epitome of "whole grain." Further, my blood glucose suffered minimal effects from the small portion I was able to stomach before becoming terribly full. Was this what most of human history had experienced when eating bread?

In contrast, mass-manufactured bread today is made by removing everything which encourages fullness and blood glucose control. The product is then made even worse by the addition of high fructose corn syrup for flavor and vegetable oil for preservation on the store shelf. Voila! Today we have the worst version of something that might have been healthy for us for nearly 6,000 years!

Worse yet, even breads and refined carbohydrates which label themselves "whole wheat" are imposters. The modern technique to make "whole wheat flour" is almost identical to the process to make highly refined white flour. In fact, most flour companies simply do the identical process to make white flour but reserve a small amount of the wheat bran off to the side. After the white flour is created, bran is added back to the white flour to create a product with a soft sandy-brown color and a slightly higher fiber content. This color difference is enough to fool most of us into believing we are eating healthfully. As you will see, this small amount of bran has almost no effect on blood glucose.

Are All Carbohydrates the Same?

It has long been known that different carbohydrates have different effects on blood glucose levels. A vegetable, for example, is not the same as a piece of hard candy. Although obvious, until 1981, no one had created a system to quantify this difference. In 1981, Drs. Wolever and Jenkins created a ranking system comparing how quickly 50 grams of carbohydrates in different foods raise blood-glucose levels. They called this system the glycemic index. The glycemic index gives glucose a numerical ranking of 100 for its potency in raising blood glucose, then compares other foods against this numerical value. For example, glucose is a 100, but 50 grams of broccoli is given a 15. This means broccoli raises blood glucose one-sixth as quickly as glucose. The Glycemic Index has long been used by endocrinologists to help educate their diabetic patients on which foods will minimally or maximally affect their blood glucose levels.

The Glycemic Index, certainly relevant for a diabetic, is also extremely relevant for any modern American trying to heal their insulin resistance and obesity. Diabetics, more than anyone else on earth, are concerned with their blood glucose. But every person who struggles with weight should be equally concerned with the glucose elevating effects of foods in their diet. The obese individual must fight against insulin response in the same way a diabetic fights to keep his or her blood sugar normal.

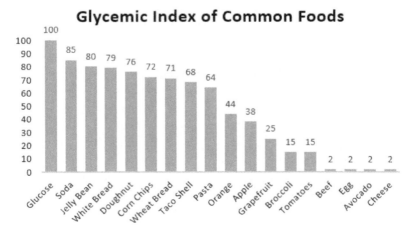

As you can see above, some foods correlate with a greater blood glucose rise, while other foods are more minimal in their effect. Both white bread and "whole-wheat" bread are almost identical in their glycemic effect on blood sugar. It is the same with white pasta versus whole wheat pasta. They both raise blood sugar very quickly, almost mimicking table sugar in their effect on the body. Foods with higher fiber content, however, have a much more muted effect. Notice the right side of the chart, in which foods designed by God are represented.

Today many diets have labeled carbohydrates as pure evil. You are told to avoid them at all costs. But when looking at this chart, we notice something very important. The foods which God made for you, despite being high in carbohydrate content, cause very minimal effects on blood glucose, and subsequently, on insulin levels in the body. Carbohydrates are not evil, nor are they solely responsible for our obesity epidemic. But as you can see, refined carbohydrates are a different beast.

From here out, we will refer to products containing the cocaine-like refined white and wheat flour as "refined carbohydrates." These are the primary carbohydrates that our society enjoys today (such as bread, pasta, tortillas, processed cereals, etc.). They are essentially all huge helpings of sugar! These products, eaten throughout the day, cause a never-ending insulin response from the body in an attempt to maintain normal blood glucose. This leads to insulin resistance, even higher insulin levels, and ultimately, obesity.

Fiber is the missing ingredient, stripped by corporations from our food, causing once harmless food products to become empty, destructive calories.

What the heck is Fiber, anyway?

Fiber is incredibly important. But what is fiber, anyway? Fiber is the portion of food, usually carbohydrate, that the body cannot digest. The chemical varieties of fiber are various, including Lignin, Cellulose, Beta-Glucans, Hemicelluloses, Pectins, Gums, Inulin, Oligofructose, and Resistant Starch.

Fiber comes in two forms: Soluble and Insoluble. This classification is based on whether the fiber itself can dissolve in water. Insoluble fiber is found primarily in the bran layers of cereal grains, whereas soluble fiber is found in foods such oats and oatmeal, legumes (peas, beans, lentils), barley, fruits, and vegetables.

Fiber can also be classified as fermentable or non-fermentable, based on whether the intestinal bacteria of the colon are able to digest the fiber on your behalf. Some examples of fermentable fiber are oats and barley, as well as fruit and vegetables. Nonfermentable fibers include Cereal fibers that are rich in cellulose, such as wheat bran. These are relatively resistant to bacterial fermentation.

Cellulose, for example, is the fiber found in tree bark. Unless you are a termite, your body has no way to break cellulose down and use it for calories. Likewise, your body has almost no mechanism to extract calories from any of these forms of fiber. Your body can obtain a very small number of calories from some "fermentable" fibers, but only after bacteria in your large intestine "ferment" them, doing the real work of digestion for you.

Fiber generally moves through the intestinal tract very quickly until it is partially digested by healthy bacteria in your large intestine, and then excreted into the world. But along the way, it has some fascinating and amazing effects.

Fiber the Great Filler

Firstly, fiber increases your feeling of fullness. Soluble fiber expands, almost like a gel as you eat it. Remember I said God didn't forget about carbohydrates? Soluble fiber is present mainly in fruits and vegetables. As you eat them, they expand in your stomach and intestines, giving your brain a strong fullness signal.

A 2017 study evaluated the "fullness" sensation induced by different carbohydrates. The researchers showed that carbohydrates with fiber created a sense of fullness significantly sooner than carbohydrates without fiber. The subjects of the study who ate large amounts of fiber-laden carbohydrates also reported decreased hunger over the following 4 hours. When your stomach is full of fiber, Ghrelin (the hunger hormone) decreases, and your hunger essentially shuts off.

Fiber the Great Mover

Next, fiber moves food along your digestive tract faster. No doubt, you have experienced this effect yourself. Anyone who has had a meal high in fiber knows to keep a bathroom close over the next few hours. Fiber is in the business of moving things through your bowels, and it does its job with gusto!

In a 1981 study, food motility through the GI tract was found to be anywhere from 50% to 900% faster when foods with high amounts of fiber were eaten. Quick indeed!

Importantly, most of the calories you eat are absorbed in a part of your intestines known as the proximal duodenum. Food is initially digested by stomach acid, then moves to the proximal duodenum, where the bulk of calories and nutrients are absorbed. Duodenum is Greek for "12", as early physicians noted this part of the intestine was roughly 12 finger-widths long.

Fiber is fascinating in that it moves food so quickly through the duodenum that the body barely has a chance to digest and absorb calories.

In modern medicine, surgeons perform a procedure known as a gastric bypass. During a gastric bypass, the stomach of an extremely obese individual is cut down to a smaller size, while at the same time the surgeon redirects the outlet of the stomach from the duodenum to a point further along the small intestine, usually at the jejunum. This forms a traffic detour of food "bypassing" the majority of the small intestine.

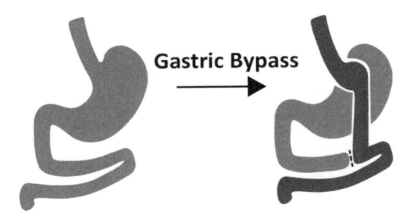

Human calorie absorption in the GI tract comes mainly from the small intestine, so the surgical recipient gets two benefits. Firstly, they have a smaller stomach, so they feel fuller sooner. Second, the food they eat skips the majority of the small intestine, and so their body cannot extract as many calories from their food. These two effects lead to profound weight loss.

The amazing thing is that God designed the human body to have the same effect as a gastric bypass simply from eating the foods which He designed. Soluble fiber swells in the stomach causing a natural fullness sensation, and then, as we have all experienced when eating high fiber foods, fibrous food moves so quickly along your small intestine that your body barely has time to extract calories before leaving the small intestine. Essentially the same effect as a gastric bypass surgery - without the pain and complications!

Fiber the Blood Glucose Reducer

By decreasing the time food spends in the heavy absorption area of the intestinal tract, fiber simply does not allow glucose to be absorbed as quickly as refined carbohydrates. Fiber "gets in the way" of the normal operations of the proximal duodenum, as well as the small intestine as a whole. By acting like a "blocker" for carbohydrate absorption, fiber stops blood glucose levels from rising quickly, as they would after the ingestion of candy, crackers, or white bread.

When your blood glucose rises, your body responds by increasing your body's insulin production and serum insulin levels. Insulin, as we will discuss further, is the single greatest hormone contributing to weight gain and the maintenance of body fat. Fiber stops this system overload of the weight-gain hormone.

Diabetics like myself have been studied at length for the effects of blood glucose control and insulin levels after eating meals heavy in fiber. The findings are wonderful. In almost all studies, blood glucose control was better and more easily maintained with a fiber-rich diet. Insulin levels were likewise decreased after fibrous meals when compared to meals rich in refined carbohydrates.

In the Nurses Health Studies I and II, participants who ate a diet rich in fiber significantly decreased their rate of type 2 diabetes. The study showed that fiber is significantly protective of insulin resistance. But this is a double-edged sword. In the same way diets rich in fiber protected against type 2 diabetes, the study showed diets rich in low-fiber refined carbohydrates increased the chance of the development of type 2 diabetes by 75%.

Likewise, the 1997 Health Professionals Follow-up Study, which followed 42,759 men over six years, showed a diet rich in refined carbohydrates and low in fiber increased risk of type diabetes of 217%!

For those of you who already have diabetes, fiber causes much more stable blood glucose levels and decreases hyperglycemia (high blood sugar). In a study done in 2017, type 2 diabetics were assigned to two groups and given standardized liquid meals, one without fiber and the other with fiber. The group receiving added fiber significantly reduced their peak blood glucose levels, as well as their peak insulin levels. There was no difference in the amount of carbohydrates or number of calories.

My own experience with fiber has been no different. As a type 1 diabetic, my body produces no insulin whatsoever. After I eat any carbohydrate, I am able to see the immediate effects on my body and to compare them. This has led to some very interesting self-experimentation. Over time, I have been able to "weed out" the foods which raise my blood glucose most and likewise try to increase my consumption of foods which cause almost no rise in blood glucose. Some foods, it turns out, do not require me to give myself any insulin whatsoever. You read that correctly: no insulin whatsoever. Imagine the weight of an individual who ate only foods which require the body to produce no insulin. Imagine the insulin sensitivity of that individual!

In my own self-experimentation, fiber-rich carbohydrates raise my blood glucose negligibly, and very, very slowly. Conversely, foods which contain high carbohydrates but minimal fiber, raise my blood glucose levels through the roof, and very rapidly! After eating such foods, I must take large amounts of exogenous (external) insulin. This causes insulin resistance within my body, as well as hormone signaling for fat storage. No thanks!

Similar to the glycemic index or glycemic load charts, let's look at common American foods in a real type 1 diabetic. Let's compare my own body's responses to 200 calories of each food. In the glycemic index, proteins and fats are not included, as they have shown minimal effect on blood glucose. I have included them to show the veracity of this claim! My chart shows the effect of 200 calories of carbohydrate, protein, and fat on a starting blood glucose of 90 mg/dl (normal blood glucose), *without* the intervention of insulin. Shown within the graph is the change in my blood glucose 2 hours after each food:

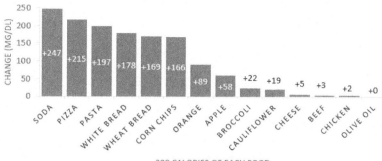

2-HOUR CHANGE IN BLOOD GLUCOSE (STARTING AT 90 MG/DL)

200 CALORIES OF EACH FOOD

Perhaps more important than any other effect which fiber offers, reduction of blood glucose and insulin requirements in the body cannot be overestimated in our goal of weight loss. The chart above, a testament to the power of fiber to negate my body's need for insulin, has huge implications on weight loss. If my body needs no insulin for certain foods, your body is the same. Likewise, if my body requires high amounts of fat-storing insulin for certain carbohydrates, yours does too! The only difference is that my insulin comes from a pharmacy bottle, and yours comes from your own pancreas.

Fiber and the Anti-Inflammatory Gut Biome

Recently, great strides have been made in the research of our "Gut Biome." The "Gut Biome" refers to the types and quantities of bacteria which live within your intestinal tract. For decades of modern medicine, these bacteria were given no thought whatsoever. In fact, any physician who mentioned the effect of intestinal bacteria were likened to naturalistic shamans, spouting woo-woo pseudo-science.

But much has changed. Medicine today fully accepts that human beings are mutualistic creatures, living in harmony with necessary and helpful "good bacteria." These bacteria reside in the intestinal tract in greater quantities than anywhere else in or on the human body.

Fiber, for its part, promotes both the healthy type of bacteria in your GI tract, as well as an "intestinal flora richness," superior in humans who eat fiber to those who do not. In today's America, we have a supposed plague of gluten allergy, irritable bowel syndrome, inflammatory bowel disease, and even the newly coined "abdominal migraine." Studies have shown, however, most "gluten allergy" is not true gluten allergy, but rather people with chronic abdominal pain searching for an answer. The answer may be much simpler.

In the human large intestine, bacteria which live almost exclusively on the digestion of fiber convert the fiber to something called "Short Chain Fatty Acids" or SCFA. These SCFA have been extensively studied, and shown to be highly anti-inflammatory. Indeed, they have been linked to decreased inflammation as well as decreased insulin resistance.

With a disrupted Gut Biome, as we would find in a diet deficient in fiber, or too rich in simple carbohydrates such as sugar and refined carbohydrate, these SCFA are diminished, and subsequently gut inflammation is increased. Could this be the cause of all of our burgeoning "belly pain"?

Without sufficient fiber on which to subsist, bacteria have been shown to eat the mucin layer of your intestine. This protective mucin layer is a healthy and normal barrier between your intestinal wall and the bacteria which reside in your GI tract. It is usually left alone by bacteria, but when the diet is deficient in fiber, the bacteria begin to eat it. This mucin layer then becomes thin and ragged, allowing bacteria to interact with the wall of the intestine.

At the intestinal wall, the bacteria come in contact with your body's immune cells, setting off inflammatory responses both in the GI tract and throughout the entire body. The cells of your intestinal tract, under the duress of severe inflammation, begin to destabilize and leak. This leads to inflammatory signals entering your bloodstream and contributing to whole-body inflammation. This is still theoretical medicine, but nevertheless the studies so far are fascinating. At present, this hypothesis for our society's increasing abdominal pain is being referred to as "Leaky Gut Syndrome."

Could this be responsible for the huge uptick in stomach aches, mock-gluten allergy, and newly coined "irritable bowel syndrome" which we are now seeing? Could a whole generation of stomach pain actually be caused by "Leaky Gut Syndrome"? I think it just might!

Worse yet, we know that inflammation causes increased insulin resistance, which in turn leads to obesity. Are we denying SCFA's through our diet, which inadvertently leads us to diabetes and obesity?

A 2007 study performed on mice showed the effects of an inflammatory chemical, LPS, which is secreted by "bad" bacteria of the gastrointestinal tract. These bacteria increase in the absence of fiber. The study showed LPS increased both insulin and leptin (a hormone we will discuss further) resistance. Likewise, a 2008 study examined the effects of tampering with intestinal bacteria in mice through antibiotics. The mice were fed antibiotics in an effort to change their intestinal microbiome. The researchers found that changes in the gut microbiota (bacteria) reduced glucose tolerance, increased insulin levels, and increased body fat.

In 2016, researchers showed that the reverse is also true in mice. Giving mice high fiber content, in an effort to protect gut bacteria, provided protection against hormonal resistance. Their results suggested that fiber may be beneficial against excess body weight, insulin resistance, and elevated blood lipids (cholesterol levels).

Where is All the Fiber?

If fiber is so amazing, why is it in *none* of our foods? The answer is simple. Since the invention of frozen and processed foods in the late 1950s, fiber *had* to be removed. You see, fiber doesn't freeze or store well when mixed with other foods. As fiber freezes, it expands. The expansion of fiber crystals leads to the destruction of the structure and texture of the surrounding food. If too much fiber is left in a processed food, the food will be destroyed during freezing and transport. Once thawed and placed on a store shelf, the person who buys this destroyed food would spit it out and never give that brand another chance!

Sure, you can freeze a bag of broccoli, but to leave the fiber in a processed, factory-churned food, such as a microwave dinner, would never work. Food companies are very much aware that any fiber left in their foods will expand when frozen, destroying many of the food particles in the rest of their food and leading to horrible taste. So, what do they do? They strip it out, and in its place, they usually add more sugar.

But TV dinners and classic frozen foods are not the only foods which are frozen in their life-cycle. Most foods in modern America are shipped great distances. Most are frozen at some point in their production process in order to preserve them for the trip. This means that almost all American processed foods must have fiber removed, or risk destroying their taste.

In place of a product which has a chance to fill you up, keep your bowel movements regular, and move food quickly and efficiently through your system, we now have foods which offer no satiety, increase blood sugar and insulin levels, and often leave you hungrier than before.

Conclusion

Fiber is incredibly important. It is the final piece of the puzzle when discussing what has changed in our food since the 1960s. Since the 1960s, we have added sugar to everything, replaced healthy fat with unnatural fat, and stripped out any chance of feeling full by removing fiber. The result? We are the fattest human beings this world has ever known! Likewise, we are all insulin resistant and hormonally imbalanced. This leads us to rule #3:

Rule #3: I will not eat refined carbohydrates. I will only eat carbohydrates which are naturally rich in fiber and minimally affect my blood glucose. (We will discuss exactly which carbohydrate-rich foods are safe to eat later).

In the next section, we will look at how the hormones in the body control your weight. Since the 1960s we have been tampering with these hormones. We have reset our biological weight-thermostats to "HIGH," and didn't even know we were doing it!

Section III

Our Disrupted Hormones

CHAPTER 7: INSULIN AND GLUCAGON, THE MASTER FAT HORMONES

Who's the Boss?

We have discussed the changes to the American diet since the 1960s, but larger questions remain. How do these foods change the hormones within our bodies and lead to weight gain? What are the major hormones responsible? Which hormone, exactly, is in charge?

Beyond storing calories, the body also has the ability to convert excess calories into heat, or to burn the calories for pure energy, and release the excess as carbon dioxide. Calories can be literally burned or breathed off, without ever being stored. No modern physician will tell you this at your appointment! The question then becomes: what tells the body to store calories, versus simply wasting them in your breath?

Caloric Wasting

Breathing off or burning excess calories for heat is called "caloric wasting." In medicine, we see this when we overfeed patients in the hospital who cannot feed themselves. When a patient is in a coma, they are often fed intravenously for the first few days. This means all of their nutrition goes straight into their veins from a product called "TPN" or "Total Parenteral Nutrition." Parenteral means "around the intestinal tract," and refers to the fact that we are going around their normal system to give calories.

These patients give us a unique window into overfeeding. What happens when we accidentally miscalculate the required calories for these comatose patients? Does their body immediately start storing the excess calories as fat? After all, modern science would tell you that every calorie you eat in excess of the calories you burn is stored as extra weight. However, in such a scenario, we see the opposite. These patients typically raise their body-heat to fever levels as they burn unneeded calories. Likewise, the respiratory rate of these patients increases to allow more carbon dioxide to be breathed off. Like a well-tuned machine, their bodies reject the sudden increase in calories, and simply waste them as heat and carbon dioxide.

Since fat cannot be both deposited and breathed off at the same time, it stands to reason that the body has a mechanism to direct excess calories to be "wasted" rather than stored.

A study done in 1999 showed this. The researchers studied comatose patients in the intensive care unit who had been administered excessive intravenous glucose loads greater than 4 mg per kg of body weight per minute. In these patients, researchers witnessed both thermogenic response (increased heat) as well as additional carbon dioxide respiration. Both the heat generation as well as the increase in carbon dioxide correlated to levels above the patient's resting energy expenditure. In other words, every calorie the body didn't need, it wasted. They noted this effect was enhanced in patients with the greatest stress response. This makes perfect sense, as we will discuss later.

Similarly, a study done in 1995 examined the hormonal response of weight loss and weight gain in 41 subjects. The study was very clever. In the first group, they took 23 subjects who had never been obese and increased their body weight by 10% through increased feeding over several weeks. The second group, consisting of 18 obese participants, was placed on a calorie restriction diet and had a decrease in body weight of 10%. As both groups had seen a 10% body weight change, the researchers then studied their resting metabolism, as well as their thermic (heat generation) effect after feeding.

In the group which started as obese, after losing 10% of body weight, resting metabolism **decreased** by 500-600 calories per day. Heat generation was virtually non-existent. However, in the group which started at normal weight, after gaining 10% of body weight, resting metabolism **increased** by nearly 700 calories per day. Of these 700 calories, approximately 400 calories were wasted as heat.

Clearly, the body has a mechanism in place to help us maintain our weight. The patients who had recently gained weight, like the overfed comatose patients given TPN, had a set mechanism within their body, which decided "that's too much." Their bodies subsequently directed calories to be wasted. Conversely, the patients who had recently lost weight, were in a full "store it all!" mode, desperately trying to preserve every calorie which they ate.

What directs the body on how to use our calories? And if we can figure out which hormones are in control, can we hijack and direct their signals in our own body?

I personally used the control of hormones to lose over 116 lbs., almost effortlessly, and have made it my mission to teach everyone how to do so. I **know** that once you wrestle control of these hormones from the horrible foods we have begun to eat since the 1970s, you will lose weight effortlessly, without any feelings of irritability, without any sensation of starvation, and without any difficulty whatsoever.

The First Master Hormone: Insulin

The first and arguably the most important hormone related to body weight is insulin. In the world of fat storage and metabolism, insulin is the absolute king. But what is insulin, exactly? From what mechanisms does it derive its power?

The textbook primary action of insulin is "An anabolic hormone created by the pancreas which stimulates glucose uptake in muscle and adipocytes via translocation of GLUT receptor vesicles to the plasma membrane." These are fancy words! But what do they mean in plain English? Let me try to simplify it.

When you eat, food is digested into single units of each macronutrient: fat, protein, and carbohydrate. These individual sub-units of each macronutrient are fatty acids, amino acids, and glucose, respectively. Both polysaccharides (from carbohydrate) and amino acids (from protein) can be broken down or converted to glucose.

Your body loves glucose. It is the primary currency of the body's energy. During times of feeding, almost all energy transactions throughout the body take place in the currency of glucose. But the body has a problem. Glucose cannot passively cross the membrane of a cell. Each cell is "locked" to glucose. Until the cell is "unlocked," no glucose can enter, and so glucose remains in the bloodstream as "blood glucose" or "blood sugar."

To get around this "locked cell," the body has a channel, or doorway, through which glucose can enter. But it can't just leave this door open all the time. If it did, some cells would take more than their share of glucose. Imbalances would occur everywhere. You would quickly drain all of the glucose out of your bloodstream, possibly leaving your brain without its portion. This would lead to seizures and death.

Therefore, this door also needs a lock. In a normal state, the glucose door on each cell stays locked until the key arrives. This key is called insulin. Insulin acts like a key on the locked glucose door of each cell. When insulin shows up, it unlocks the glucose channel (the glucose door), and glucose is allowed to enter the cell to be used as energy or stored as fat.

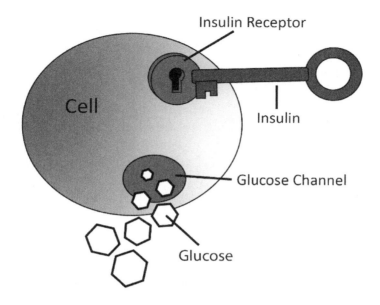

In medical school, most physicians are taught about the regulation of blood glucose by insulin. We are not, however, taught about insulin's importance in obesity. Every American should understand their body's insulin, not just the diabetics. As important as blood glucose control is, that is only a fraction of insulin's job within the body.

Insulin is also anabolic, which means "pro-growth." Anabolism (anabolic), in the context of your body, means you are in a state of building up or storing. Insulin, by its very nature, promotes the building of fat stores, the building of muscle, and strong resistance to the opposite. If we think of insulin like a personality in a story, insulin is the character who wants to hoard, hoard, hoard, and never let a single calorie be wasted. Insulin is the Ebenezer Scrooge of hormones. Insulin commands the entire body: "Do not spend a dime! All must be saved, kept, and used to build up our ever-increasing wealth of calories!" What this translates to for the modern human is: "Get fatter! We must be rich in stored calories!"

Insulin is so pro-growth that professional weight lifters have been known to use injections of insulin, at great peril to their health, to promote muscle mass increases. It is not uncommon for professional body-builders to obtain insulin on the black market and to take injections before protein-loading and glucose-loading, all in an effort to stimulate anabolic growth.

Glucagon: The Anti-Insulin

Glucagon, however, is the nemesis of insulin. Glucagon is a very different hormone. If insulin is Ebenezer Scrooge, glucagon would be the reckless spendthrift in our story, blowing through savings like there was no tomorrow! Glucagon cackles as he burns 100-dollar bills for warmth. With a mischievous grin on his face, glucagon sets fire to his own house, dancing as it burns. Glucagon's mantra is "Tear it all down. Spend it all!" Glucagon is catabolic.

Catabolism in the body is the state of "tearing-down" or, in the case of fat, burning down. Catabolism results in loss of fat stores, and a propensity to use calories for anything *but* fat storage. Glucagon directs the body to burn calories off as heat or to excrete them in the breath or urine as ketones rather than to store them. To glucagon, storage is the absolute worst idea the body could have. As overweight individuals, we love glucagon!

Both insulin and glucagon are made by the body in the pancreas. In fact, they are made side by side in the pancreas in cells called beta and alpha cells (respectively). Next door neighbors they may be, but they are mortal enemies. In all ways, they are opposed to each other. In the body, God loves balance, and it is the balance of these two characters which controls, in almost every way, the fat you either burn or deposit daily. When insulin dominates, you store fat. When glucagon dominates, fat is burned.

To prove that the ratio of insulin and glucagon in your body controls your weight, we need to look at some examples of when the body's normal function goes awry. As we mentioned in chapter 2, sometimes the best way to evaluate the normal function of a hormone within the body is to look at what happens when it breaks.

Type 1 Diabetes

Diabetes was first recorded in ancient Egypt, noted for the

symptoms of frequent urination and extreme weight loss. Later, in ancient Greece, diabetes was further described by the physician Aretus, who named the disease diabainein, which means "a siphon." This referred to the fact that diabetics typically urinated in great quantities, like water through a siphon. This still happens today, as the increased urination is due to the osmotic effect (pulling of water) as water follows high glucose concentrations into the urine.

Prior to 1922, type 1 diabetes was fatal. In 1921 Physician Frederick Banting and his medical student assistant, Charles H. Best, discovered the hormone insulin in the pancreatic extracts of dogs. On July 30, 1921, they injected this newly discovered hormone into a diabetic dog and found that it effectively lowered the dog's blood glucose levels to normal.

Before 1922, a newly diagnosed type 1 diabetic had no options whatsoever to obtain insulin. Since we know what insulin does in the body, can you guess what happened to a young child who had no endogenous insulin (insulin created by their body?). Remember, insulin is the master storage hormone, directing fat storage, and guarding against the burning of fat. It normally fights the action of glucagon, which prefers *no* fat storage. With this in mind, what would happen if you removed all insulin from the body? Well, type 1 diabetes tells us exactly what would happen.

Typically, when a child develops type 1 diabetes, one of the first signs is increased thirst, as well as increased urination. Some children, who have never wet the bed in their life, will begin to rise from sleep to get a glass of water, return to bed and immediately urinate in their sleep. Obviously, this causes alarm bells to go off in the minds of the parents.

Personally, at age 9, I began to urinate and thirst constantly. My vision became blurred. I began to beg for more to drink when at home or in restaurants. One night at a restaurant, after asking for my 9th glass of water, the waiter joked with my father that I should forget the water and just get hooked to an IV. How right he was!

But this is not the greatest symptom or sign of type 1 diabetes.

Without exception, the most disturbing sign is weight loss. Type 1 diabetics, often starting at a normal weight, become skeletal in appearance before their diagnosis is made. The weight loss is rapid and disturbing. Parents watch their children waste away before their eyes.

In my own case, I began at a weight of 62 pounds at age 9. This is a very normal weight and well within all current BMI charts for a 9-year-old. By the time of my diagnosis, I weighed a mere 40 pounds — the weight of a typical 5-year-old.

So disturbing is the weight loss in type 1 diabetes that the ancient Greek physician Aretus described diabetes further as, "the melting down of flesh and limbs into urine." For nearly 2000 years before diabetes was fully understood, scientists recognized that it was associated with profound weight loss and even emaciation. For much of the 20th century, this was thought to be due solely to cellular starvation.

It was believed that because the child made no insulin, insulin could not act as a key for glucose to enter the cells. Glucose, therefore, was unable to go through the "glucose door," and thus, the cells began to starve. Glucose then traffic jammed in the blood, unable to get into the cell, leading to high blood glucose levels. This, in turn, led to thirst and urination. The body, because no glucose was available, was forced to switch to fat metabolism for energy. Stores of body fat were quickly burned away, and the child starved internally, despite being fed.

Of course, this is accurate, and no modern physician would dispute this general mechanism for type 1 diabetes. However, this modern explanation does not go far enough. Cellular starvation, as an explanation for weight loss, neglects another part of the equation. When we look at a human being's insulin and glucagon, we must also consider the balance between these two hormones. We refer to this balance as the Insulin: Glucagon Ratio. That is to say, the ratio of balance between both insulin and glucagon.

Because the body sees both insulin and glucagon regularly, the actions each hormone inspires is regulated not by the hormone itself, but by the balance between the two. Your body evaluates which hormone predominates, and on that basis makes its hormonal decision. A lack of either hormone, as in the case of type 1 diabetes, creates a relative *infinite* surplus of the other hormone. In other words, if there is 0 insulin, the respective amount of *glucagon is infinite*.

$$\frac{\text{Glucagon}}{\text{Insulin (0)}} = \infty \quad \text{Infinite Glucagon}$$

When we hold to our analogy of Ebenezer Scrooge (insulin) vs. the Mad Spendthrift (glucagon), type 1 diabetes is a scenario in which Ebenezer Scrooge is absent within the story. The Mad Spendthrift reigns, doing as he pleases with all the body's fat storage. Catabolism (burning down) is the only active hormonal mechanism, while anabolism (building up) is completely absent. This is exactly what we find in undiagnosed type 1 diabetics.

As awful as type 1 diabetes is, we can learn much from this process. As discussed above, the lack of insulin causes exactly the response we would expect. The master hormone becomes glucagon, and the ratio tips in glucagon's favor toward a hormonal state in which fat is loaded up by the handful, and burned off as rapidly as possible. The body becomes a fat-burning machine, irrespective of any other input.

Today we even have a new issue among type 1 diabetics who have realized the potency of weight loss while not under the effect of insulin. The phenomenon has been coined "Diabulimia" and refers to diabetics who willingly withhold their insulin to promote weight loss. Does it work? You bet. Is it healthy? Heck, no.

While I can tell you from experience that an infinite glucagon ratio is not fun, we can harness the power of this hormonal balance to lose weight safely and effectively, the way our body was intended. In America today, we live in a state where our hormonal Ebenezer

Scrooge has been allowed to reign unhindered. We save, save, save, and store calories, without ever letting our Mad Spendthrift, glucagon, have any say.

Modern Americans keep glucagon locked deep in the basement, tied up and gagged. Prior generations, however, lived in a balance between insulin and glucagon. At times they stored calories; at other times they burned them feverishly. Due to the modern American diet, we have lost access to our own hormonal balance, handed the keys to insulin, and destroyed our body's ability to maintain a normal weight through the power of glucagon.

Insulin:Glucagon Ratio – The Absolute Key to Weight Loss

If the ratio of insulin to glucagon is the master signal instructing our body on whether to gain fat or, likewise, whether to shed it, what influence can our food choices and dietary actions have on this ratio? It turns out that control of this ratio is entirely in our hands.

In the 1960s and 1970s, perhaps the most important studies ever done concerning weight loss were performed. During the studies, famed endocrinologist Robert Unger and a team of researchers evaluated the insulin to glucagon ratio of dogs under different dietary conditions.

In the first group of dogs, measurements of insulin and glucagon were taken after 12 hours of fasting. During this time, they found the insulin to glucagon ratio to be roughly 0.8. This means for every one insulin molecule, there were nearly two glucagon molecules. Glucagon was the predominant hormone.

What would we expect during such times? What effects would a ratio consisting of an elevated glucagon and relatively low insulin create? In such patients, we see no new fat creation or fat storage. *The body is unable to store fat*. At the same time, body fat is directed to be torn down for energy.

After fasting, the canine subjects were then fed each macronutrient, in turn, to examine its effect. During IV infusion of glucose, the ratio of insulin to glucagon increased to roughly 4.0. This is the same general ratio of insulin to glucagon we find in modern Americans. This represents four insulin molecules to every one glucagon molecule. This is a fat-storage ratio.

Next, researchers infused fatty acids. After the infusion of pure fat, the increase of the ratio was far lower, roughly at 1.3. This ratio of 1.3 insulin to 1 glucagon essentially means the body is neutral, neither storing fat nor burning it.

Most surprisingly, after the consumption of pure protein, the ratio *decreased* from 0.8 to 0.5. ***This cannot be overstated***. After infusing a load of pure amino acids (protein), the canines not only maintained an elevated glucagon ratio, but the ratio was *even better* than during fasting. At 0.5 insulin to every 1.0 of glucagon, their bodies continued to burn fat even after obtaining calories!

As the above study shows, glucose (carbohydrate) is the greatest inducer of a high insulin to glucagon ratio. This makes sense, as the body must produce insulin to utilize the "key" effect of insulin and allow the entry of the glucose, from carbohydrate-rich foods, into the cells. The other macronutrients, fat and protein, are essentially neutral or beneficial (respectively) to the insulin: glucagon ratio. What might the diet of a society such as America, in which every food contains added sugar, do to this ratio?

To Store or Not to Store: The Ratio's Decision

Under differing ratios of insulin to glucagon, each macronutrient is then utilized by the body differently. Let's look at how the body processes fat, protein, and carbohydrate under the direction of a high insulin to glucagon ratio versus a low insulin to glucagon ratio.

Insulin to Glucagon Ratio > 1.0 (High Insulin)

Dietary Fat: Under a high insulin ratio, the dietary fat you eat is taken up by the fat cells and added to fat stores. Fat stores are often composed of the exact fats eaten by the individual in this circumstance. This is seen in overfed cows, whose adipose tissue makeup resembles the corn oil eaten prior to slaughter.

Dietary Protein: High insulin to glucagon ratio promotes the breakdown of the individual molecules of protein, called amino acids, into pyruvate molecules. Pyruvate molecules are then converted to acetyl-CoA and ultimately linked together into a fatty acid chain. This fatty acid is then transported to the fat tissue of the body, where it is stored.

Dietary Carbohydrate: Dietary carbohydrate breaks down to individual molecules of glucose (except in the case of fructose). High I:G (insuling:glucagon) ratio promotes the storage of glycogen (glucose storage), followed by the conversion of glucose molecules into acetyl-CoA and subsequently, fatty acid. This fatty acid is likewise directed to be stored on the body as excess fat.

Insulin to Glucagon Ratio < 1.0 (Low Insulin)

Dietary Fat: Under a low I:G ratio, dietary fat is either taken up directly by hungry cells to be used as energy or converted to ketones in the liver. These ketones are then used by the body for energy. Some of these ketone molecules are wasted in the urine or breath, leading to calorie loss. Fat is directed to the skeletal muscle and other body tissue to be burned in the mitochondria for energy, or as heat. This again leads to the destruction of ingested calories.

Dietary Protein: Under the direction of a low I:G ratio, 36% of dietary protein is used to build glucose. Proteins are broken down into their individual unit of amino acids, which are then converted, via a biochemical pathway known as gluconeogenesis, to glucose. This glucose is then used as energy for the brain (which will only accept a maximum of 67% ketones and requires at least 33% glucose), the red blood cells (which cannot use ketones), or the body tissue in general.

Under these conditions, amino acids are not stored as fat. We find that only a third of dietary protein can be used to create glucose. The remaining amino acids are taken up by skeletal muscle cells, as well as other tissue cells, to be directed into protein creation. As you will see later in this book, muscle continues to be created and maintained even during times of high glucagon, or in times of fasting.

Dietary Carbohydrate: Under the influence of low insulin to glucagon, carbohydrate is directed to the TCA cycle, where it is burned for energy. It is not directed to fat storage. However, high carbohydrate loads generally do not allow for a low insulin state, as insulin responds most quickly and readily to carbohydrate loads.

The important point: Under the influence of high insulin and low glucagon, *every* macronutrient is eventually converted to fat. Conversely, under the influence of low insulin and high glucagon, *none* of the macronutrients are directed to fat storage. This, my friends, is the key to weight loss.

Type 2 Diabetes and Too Much Insulin

We have discussed the disease scenario of a type 1 diabetic, in which a person has little or no insulin, and has a relatively high glucagon level. This scenario leads to extreme weight loss. But what about the situation in which the person has too much insulin? What would you expect that individual's body to look like? How about their fat-burning metabolism? Luckily, we have seen those effects too.

In type 2 diabetes, the disease of diabetes is caused by a very different mechanism than that of the type 1 counterpart. Rather than resulting from an immune attack on beta cells, the type 2 diabetic is a product of diet. The typical type 2 diabetic has, through years of poor diet, developed insulin resistance.

Insulin resistance results from years of pancreatic overload. Over multiple decades, the pancreas, fighting a diet high in refined carbohydrates and sugar, has been overproducing insulin to try and keep blood glucose normal despite constant assault by high glucose loads. Think of it this way: if one of the main jobs of insulin is to keep your blood sugar levels normal, and all you eat is cake, do you think the pancreas will work harder to create insulin and keep your blood sugar down? Of course, it will! And unfortunately, the

American diet is very close to all cake! This is exactly what we see in our type 2 diabetic patients.

In type 2 diabetes, the pancreas is a little hero, fighting constantly to keep blood sugar normal despite a diet rich in sugary foods. But eventually, the body is exposed to too much insulin. The body, as it does with any drug or other chemical, becomes "used-to" or desensitized to insulin. In the same way a drug addict needs higher and higher amounts of narcotic to "get their fix," the body requires higher and higher insulin to produce the same blood glucose control.

The type 2 diabetic's blood glucose rises as insulin becomes less effective, and so the pancreas simply tries to create more insulin. A typical type 2 diabetic may have serum (blood) insulin levels 4-5 times higher than a non-diabetic counterpart. As the body produces ever higher amounts of insulin to control blood glucose, what do you think happens to the type 2 diabetic's Insulin to Glucagon ratio? It shoots to the moon! Glucagon, which does not increase in proportion to insulin, is left in the dust!

Though insulin is only being created by the pancreas to try and keep blood glucose levels normal, it has another unintended consequence. It promotes fat. Though the body *can* become desensitized to the glucose regulating effects of insulin, it *cannot* become desensitized to the fat storage effects. So, the person with insulin resistance and a 4 times increased insulin level has poor glucose control but gains weight very efficiently.

If this is true, what would we expect our typical type 2 diabetic to look like? We would expect an overweight individual, with elevated blood glucose levels. Is that typical? In fact, it is textbook. This is the exact picture of the average American type 2 diabetic.

And it gets worse. Body fat, due to its highly inflammatory nature, further contributes to insulin resistance. The fat on your body causes you to become even less sensitive to insulin, so the spiral into madness continues. As the type 2 diabetic gets fatter, their poor pancreas has an *even harder* time controlling blood glucose levels, so it creates more insulin to try to keep up. This does little for blood sugar, but causes even more hormonal signaling for weight gain. This results in *even more* increased fat storage, weight gain, and then *even further* insulin resistance.

And yet it gets even worse. The type 2 diabetic's physician, noting elevated blood glucose levels, begins the patient on medications such as sulfonylureas, which direct the pancreas to *work harder* and secrete even more insulin. The poor pancreas, already an overheated smoking engine, is told to ramp up its rpm and go faster! This leads to yet higher insulin levels, a higher insulin to glucagon ratio, higher insulin resistance, and even higher weight gain. The cycle continues.

At some point, the pancreas simply cannot keep up. It was a valiant soldier, chasing your blood glucose levels for decades, but like a mistreated heart, at some point, it just succumbs to the strain under which the type 2 diabetic body has placed it.

When this happens, the type 2 diabetic typically presents to the ER or doctor's office with symptoms which result from very elevated blood glucose. In my own practice, these symptoms are typically increased urination, increased thirst, blurred vision, and headache. At this point, labs are drawn which reveal a blood glucose of 400-500 mg/dl (normal < 120 mg/dl). What does the physician do now? Well, there is only one thing left to do: we start the patient on insulin shots.

Since the pancreas has failed, insulin must now come from an exogenous source (outside the body), and so the patient is prescribed insulin injections. There is now no limit to the amount of insulin the individual can take! 3,000 units a month? 10,000 units a month? 20,000 units a month? Why not?

Likewise, there is no limit to how high modern medicine can push the patient's insulin to glucagon ratio, and no limit to how fat we can direct their body to become. Glucagon doesn't stand a chance.

Insulin Causes Weight Gain

If the premise of this book is true, that high insulin levels lead to weight gain, can we prove this from studies? Indeed, we can.

In the 1998 UKPDS (UK Prospective Diabetes Study), 3,867 newly diagnosed patients with type 2 diabetes were assigned to aggressive treatment with insulin, versus a group in which dietary changes, rather than insulin, were implemented. The group receiving aggressive insulin therapy had better glucose control, but what happened to their weight? It increased by 30%, directly as a result of intensive insulin therapy.

A 2001 study similarly evaluated type 1 diabetics in the setting of aggressive insulin therapy. The study compared those diabetics receiving only 1-2 injections of insulin per day, under conventional therapy, with subjects receiving multiple frequent daily injections. The participants' weights were measured at baseline and at annual visits for 6 years. The group treated aggressively with frequent insulin injections, over 6 years, gained 15% of body weight, all as fatty tissue. Both groups took insulin throughout the study. The aggressive group simply took more. These results show the powerful effects of taking *slightly* more insulin.

A further 2017 study followed 40 type 2 diabetic patients over 12 months after beginning insulin therapy. The average weight gain was 10 - 15 pounds in the first year. Likewise, a 2016 study followed 340 type 2 diabetics over the first year of insulin therapy. Their findings were similar, with roughly 10 pounds of pure body fat gained over the first 12 months of insulin therapy.

These studies show that insulin directly correlates to excessive weight gain. The irony, of course, is that the doctors are trying to treat the blood glucose of these patients, but are continuing a spiraling cycle of further weight gain, further insulin resistance, and higher insulin doses. It is a dangerous and never-ending cycle.

Likewise, in type 1 diabetics, insulin is known to cause the same weight gain. After insulin became available, the emaciated, sickly type 1 diabetics quickly became "chunky kids," all through the effect of insulin's potent fat storage mechanics. I gained roughly 40 lbs. after starting on insulin as a child. I went from being the near-skeletal sickly kid to being the husky kid. Is this typical for type 1 diabetics? Absolutely.

In a 2004 study, type 1 diabetics were followed for 18 years after beginning insulin therapy. At baseline, very few participants were overweight or obese. In the 18 years of the study, the number of overweight study participants increased by 47%, while the number of obese increased by 700%.

In America, We Are All Type 2 Diabetic

If you are not yet type 2 diabetic, you may soon become one. Recent studies have shown that even among the "thin" people in developed nations eating the standard modern diet, type 2 diabetes is on the rise.

As we discussed in chapter 2, it has recently been discovered that human beings may be outwardly thin but inwardly obese, a state known as TOFI or "thin outside, fat inside." The study revealed high levels of visceral organ fat, even among the thin human beings who currently eat our horrendous American diet. Though you may appear relatively normal weight, your body may be laden with this organ fat, deposited over years of unhealthy American eating. It is this fat which, over multiple studies, has been shown to have the highest correlation to insulin resistance and type 2 diabetes. And you may not even know you have it!

Visceral fat is responsible for the highest "pre-diabetic" levels ever recorded. It is estimated that in a country of 325 million Americans, 84 million of us are bordering on diabetes. That is a whopping 25%. 30 million, or 10%, are already diagnosed with the disease. This is unbelievable. 114 million people are struggling with elevated blood glucose and insulin resistance. Contrast this to the 1960s, in which less than 2% had diabetes, and only 5% showed signs of pre-diabetes. I submit to you that *everyone* in America is on the path to diabetes due to the unbelievable dietary changes which we outlined in the first section of this book. If even our thin people are diabetic and on the path toward the spiral of insulin resistance and weight gain, what can be done?

The Chicken or the Egg

There is currently a debate among modern physicians. The debate is this: does getting fat cause people to get diabetes, or does becoming diabetic cause people to get fat? In other words, which came first – the chicken or the egg?

Many modern scientists propose that over the last 50 years, Americans ate too much, exercised too little, and became fatter as a nation. This led to type 2 diabetes. The solution, therefore, is to exercise more and eat less. We see this thinking and these recommendations nearly everywhere!

These scientists likewise recommend a high carbohydrate, low saturated fat diet. Their theory is that high saturated fat intake leads to high body fat. This high body fat, in turn, leads to insulin resistance and type 2 diabetes.

But there are several problems with this theory. First, we see almost no type 2 diabetes in cultures who eat high amounts of animal meat and fats as their primary calorie source. The Inuit, a culture which relied almost exclusively on animal meat and saturated fat, had a rate of type 2 diabetes of 0.4% in the general population prior to the arrival of refined carbohydrates and sugar. Almost zero! If eating saturated fat were the cause of body fat, we would expect this rate to have been higher.

Likewise, the native Americans were historically thin, with no known type 2 diabetes, until European society began to meld with their own. The big things Europeans brought to these cultures? Refined flour and sugar. Both are extreme elevators of blood glucose and insulin resistance. Prior to the intervention of the European diet, diabetes and obesity were unknown in the native American population.

Contrast these near-zero rates of type 2 diabetes in the Inuit and Native Americans to the type 2 diabetes rate in modern America, where we have reduced our fat intake from 40% of our diet in 1960, to roughly 25% of our diet in 2019. Our type 2 diabetes rates are 35% of the general public. Something doesn't add up.

Believing, without scientific evidence, that eating saturated fat causes a person to deposit body fat makes about as much sense as believing that eating too many strawberries will turn you pink! The process is much more complex than modern medicine admits, and saturated fat is not the enemy.

The second problem with the "fat first" hypothesis was already explored in the first section of this book. The problem is that almost no one was fat before the 1970s when the "experts" recommended we drop our dietary saturated fat.

Since the dietary recommendations of the 1970s, we have seen a quadrupling in type 2 diabetes, and a quintupling of obesity. Obesity and diabetic complications are through the roof. Every scientist, no matter their belief on the true cause of our problem, now calls our obesity issue a "national epidemic." Everyone admits there is a problem. But the treatment recommended for the last 50 years has not worked.

How Our Foods Ruined Our Ratio

Insulin and Glucagon are vitally important to weight control. In today's culture, we live in a toxic waste dump of chemical foods which *all*, without exception, increase insulin resistance. Subsequently, this insulin resistance leads to higher and higher insulin to glucagon ratios, and eventually to obesity.

Let's take a quick look at the foods which have begun to predominate in American culture, and their effect on the insulin to glucagon ratio:

Sugar and Corn Syrup: Fructose (50% of sugar) and as much as 90% of High Fructose Corn Syrup, directly leads to insulin resistance and subsequently higher insulin needs. This leads to 'round-the-clock' higher Insulin to Glucagon ratios and fat storage. Corn Syrup was unknown in the human diet prior to 1973, and today is present in nearly every processed food. Likewise, sugar has quintupled its amounts in every American food, including in non-sweet products such as bread and corn chips. Sugar and Corn Syrup are present in nearly every processed food.

Poly-Unsaturated Fats (Vegetable Oils): Almost all natural saturated fats and mono-unsaturated oils have been replaced with poly-unsaturated vegetable oils. Predominant among them is soybean oil. These oils are known to increase inflammation and insulin resistance. Likewise, in mice, these chemicals are known obesogens. Since 1970, the amount of polyunsaturated fats in the American diet has increased by 1400%. These oils lead to even higher insulin levels and Insulin to Glucagon Ratios. They are present in nearly every processed food.

Refined Carbohydrates: Fiber increases insulin sensitivity and decreases insulin levels. Insulin needs are less with fibrous foods, and so insulin to glucagon levels are lower. Refined carbohydrates remove this effect by removing all fiber. This leads to carbohydrates which spike insulin quickly and maintain high insulin levels longer. Fiber has been removed from nearly every processed food.

Looking at these food changes, which began in the 1970s, one would almost think someone designed our diet to cause us to get fat and sick. Our modern American diet is so perfectly attuned to the task of increasing insulin resistance and obesity that it boggles the mind.

The Real Solution

But what if we designed a diet to keep insulin levels, and subsequently insulin resistance, to an absolute minimum? In other words, what if we do the exact opposite of what has been done to the American diet since 1970? By removing everything that increases insulin, as well as every substance shown to increase insulin resistance, we could reset the modern American's hormonal balance.

If that sounds reasonable to you, stay tuned. That is the purpose of this book. As we move forward, we will look to develop a plan based around decreasing insulin levels in your body. Our goal will be to eliminate ***everything and anything*** that increases our resistance to insulin. We will return our insulin sensitivity to its absolute highest possible level through diet, thereby decreasing the amount of insulin your body needs to use on a daily basis. This will lead to a rapid decrease in your fat storage.

Furthermore, we will find that some very other interesting hormones begin to work more efficiently when we apply this. These other hormones, which we will discuss shortly, do everything in their power to help you shed the pounds.

Rule #4: I will strive to keep my insulin levels at a minimum. This will allow glucagon to more easily become the dominant hormone, switching my body to fat metabolism. (We will discuss how to do this later!)

<u>Important Point:</u> Through the dietary changes which we will discuss in this book, I reduced my necessary insulin from 7,000 units per month down to 650 units per month. This is a 91% reduction in insulin! Because of this reduction in insulin, weight simply melted off of my body. Though you will not be able to see your own insulin levels (unless you are diabetic), know that the same thing will happen inside your body if you follow the guidelines of the Dr. Cimino Weight Loss Solution.

CHAPTER 8: **LEPTIN**

<u>Why Do I Feel Like I'm Starving?</u>

As an obese individual, I used to watch my thin friends with absolute fascination. After eating a single slice of pizza, they would claim to be full. They would refuse any further food and immediately move on to other activities. At the time, I believed their will-power was incredible. No matter how I tried to distract my mind, the pizza left uneaten would hold my attention.

The only explanation for my friend's disinterest in eating more was that they were lying about being full, and simply restraining themselves. In my heart of hearts, I believed these people were truly starving inside, forgoing any second helping of delicious pizza simply to maintain a trim figure. I believed everyone must have higher willpower than I had. But what if there is another possibility?

In the late 20th century, a hormone was discovered which completely and utterly controls both your hunger sensation, as well as your metabolism. This hormone, when not properly sensed and functional within the body, sends the human mind a "starvation signal." When harnessed properly by the body, it also functions as the most potent hunger suppressant known to man. Let's look at how science found it.

<u>Leptin Is Discovered</u>

In 1921, scientists Bailey and Bremer proved that the hypothalamus was involved in obesity in mammals. The scientists induced hypothalamic lesions in dogs, which subsequently led to profound weight gain in the animals. They were, in a sense, honing in on the way the brain may cause or restrict obesity. In 1926, the science was replicated in rats. Rats with a lesion to the hypothalamus quickly became obese after the lesion was induced.

Later, in 1949, Jackson labs identified a specific genotype (genetic makeup) in mice which caused obesity. This genetically mutated mouse became critically important for the understanding of the brain chemistry involved with obesity. Its discovery led to further research, all searching for a ***mystery hormone*** which may control metabolism and appetite. Over the last 50 years, experiments led to the identification of what science called, "A circulating factor which powerfully controls body fatness." Now you have my attention!

As subsequent research was conducted, the theory became this: after gaining body fat, the mammalian body secreted *some hormone* from *somewhere* which acted on the hypothalamus to decrease appetite and cause the mammal (usually a mouse) to walk away from all further feedings. When this gene was absent or broken, the mammal would eat almost continuously.

Interestingly, further studies showed the mice with absent or broken genes for this "factor" preferred to stay in one corner of their cage without moving. The mice tried to burn no calories from physical exertion. Normal mice, meanwhile, ate until fullness and when finished eating, began to pace their cages nearly all day. This hormone, whatever it may be, also directed the body toward or against calorie expenditure through movement!

Finally, in 1994, scientists honed in on this factor further. They described a protein hormone which they named "Leptin." Leptin, they stated, is a peptide hormone secreted by adipose tissue in proportion to its mass. In other words, it is a hormone made by the body fat of a mammal in proportion to how fat the animal is. Animals with less fat have less leptin, while animals with more body fat have significantly more.

The researchers further described that leptin circulates in the blood and acts on the hypothalamus to regulate food intake and energy expenditure. That is to say, this hormone controls how much you eat or don't eat, and how much you want to move around.

This is important! Leptin is basically an "inventory" of fat on the body. Let's use an analogy. In your mind, I want you to picture a guy with a clipboard going around the body and counting a warehouse of fat, then reporting to the hypothalamus (his boss), to tell exactly how much fat is on the body. When stores are high, leptin reports "too much fat, sir" and the boss enacts mechanisms to lose weight. When fat stores are low, leptin reports "almost out of fat, sir," and mechanisms are enacted to get fat back.

Starting with mice in whom leptin was absent, scientists attempted to reverse obesity by giving intramuscular injections of the hormone. Within 24 hours of leptin injections, the mice began to move around their cages more, eat less, and within days began to return to normal weight!

Leptin in Humans

After describing this hormone in mice, researchers went on to search for humans who might share the same genetic leptin deficiency. Researchers found a unique group of people in Turkey and India whose children often displayed strange levels of profound obesity from an early age. These children, from the day they were born, expressed nothing but extreme hunger. They acted continually as though they were being starved. The parents were unable to satisfy the child no matter how much they fed them. Throughout their first two years of life, these children quickly became obese.

The parents complained that the children "cried out at all times for food, only calming when they were actively eating." Scientists reported that the children "ate like they were starving at all times", and by age 8 weighed as much as 500 lbs. In a study done to see if the missing hormone was leptin, these children were given intra-muscular leptin shots, with stunning results. Almost overnight, the children became less interested in food, began to play and exercise normally, and in 3-4 years returned to totally normal and healthy weights for their age.

The study found that, under the influence of leptin, both activity levels and appetite changed proportionately to the hormonal injection. Without being instructed to do so, participants naturally reduced their caloric intake by 50% and increased their activity level. For the first time in their life, the hypothalamus was getting the signal that they were "too fat" and beginning its natural mechanisms to defeat this.

Perhaps most importantly, participants in this study had only a slight decrease in metabolism while losing weight. This decrease in metabolism was almost negligible when compared to typical calorie-restriction diets, in which metabolic rate can slow by 25% in the first few weeks. The researchers concluded that leptin must prevent slowing of the metabolic rate during weight loss. This makes logical sense. If the hypothalamus senses high levels of body fat, why would it try to slow your weight loss by decreasing your metabolism?

Another study, performed in 2002, demonstrated the same effect. The study found that leptin injections successfully thwarted drops in thyroid levels, as well as decreases in basal metabolic rate, which are normally seen during weight loss.

Even more encouraging, the patients treated with leptin showed increased efficiency at fat oxidation (the burning of fat) during their entire weight loss. This means that leptin likely signals the body to become better adapted to the metabolism and breakdown of fatty tissue.

Interestingly, a 2007 study also showed that appropriate leptin levels change the preferred macronutrient of the body. The study showed, over a 12-month course of leptin injections, participants primarily craved *fats*, rather than *carbohydrates*. Again, this makes sense. If the hypothalamus is trying to direct weight loss, and carbohydrates cause elevations in insulin levels, it is very logical for the hypothalamus to maintain a high glucagon level in your body by decreasing your appetite for carbohydrates. Like I have said before, God's system is amazing!

Through the findings of these studies, as well as multiple others, leptin was further defined as a hormone which:

1. Maintains elevated metabolism even during weight loss

2. Increases fat-burning capacity

3. Powerfully reduces appetite

4. Changes macronutrient cravings from carbohydrate to fat

5. Increases the desire to move or exercise

That is my kind of hormone!

Leptin Deficiency and the Hypothalamus

As scientists gained more and more data on leptin deficiency, they concluded that, because leptin was non-functional in these patients, their hypothalamus was getting a signal from their body that said, "fat stores are critically low." This, in turn, caused the hypothalamus to act as though the body was in extreme starvation, where even vital organ fat could not be maintained.

Though the patient was obese, the body perceived starvation and increased the appetite to levels which would be expected in someone on the edge of death from food deprivation. This explains the reports of the parents of leptin-deficient children who stated they could never satisfy their child. The child's brain was sending out a starvation signal!

During *true* starvation, the body will utilize several mechanisms to try to preserve calories for critical bodily functions. Humans have been shown during extreme starvation (weeks to months of no food) to decrease thyroid function and basal metabolism, to decrease immune function, and lastly to increase insulin resistance. The body is trying, desperately, to fight off starvation by decreasing caloric use and functions which it views as non-critical.

What boggled the minds of the scientists studying leptin was that all of these starvation effects were present in the leptin-deficient humans and animals. In other words, their body perceived that they were truly starving, despite super-obese weights and body mass indexes in excess of 50%! No wonder they were hungry all the time!

Leptin, in the normal human being, is supposed to give a signal to the brain that fat stores are plentiful. Yet in modern America, when we lose 10 pounds of fat, we have an overwhelming "starvation" signal, very similar to that of the patients with deficient or mutated leptin. Leptin, produced by our fatty tissue, is a potent regular of metabolism, hunger, and weight gain. A hormone produced *by* fat is meant to inhibit you from gaining *more* fat. So, what went wrong?

Then Why Are We Obese?

I know what you are thinking: If leptin is so potent a regulator of appetite and metabolism, why are we obese to begin with? Could Americans be leptin-deficient? Is that the cause of our obesity? Well, let me tell you, that was the first thing scientists thought of after discovering the hormone! What they found was a disappointment to many.

In a randomized, double-blind, placebo-controlled trial done from 1997 to 1998, leptin injections were given to obese adult study participants. Importantly, these obese adults *were not leptin-deficient*. This is the key difference. Their bodies made normal amounts and quality of the leptin hormone. In the study, 73 obese adults were studied under the effects of intramuscular leptin injections over a 20-week course. During this time, the placebo group lost no weight, as expected. The leptin-treated group, however, didn't do much better. Their average weight loss was a dismal, though not insignificant, 10 pounds (4.5 kg) over 5 months.

As you can see above, obese Americans given leptin lost very little weight. Worse, appetite remained the same, and energy expenditure (movement) did not change. So, what gives? If leptin is such a powerful hormone to stop weight gain, why did Americans without a rare mutation in their leptin hormone gain weight in the first place?

Why didn't this beautiful brain chemistry prevent their obesity?

Leptin resistance

After the failure of leptin injections in obese Americans, scientists began to look at the circulating blood levels of leptin in the average obese American and found that levels were often much higher than in non-obese counterparts. This seemed to indicate the problem was not with a deficiency in the hormone itself, but rather in the body's *sensitivity to leptin*.

In fact, scientists found that obese Americans have **tons** of leptin circulating in their blood. This leptin, created by their fat cells, reaches the hypothalamus as intended, and yet their body acts as though they are perfectly thin, with normal or even sub-normal levels of body fat. This creates a hypothalamic condition in which the body is absolutely loathe to lose any weight, and tries to maintain the obese body weight as though the person were borderline under-fed.

The cause, they postulated, was that obese humans could become leptin-resistant, in much the same way they can become insulin-resistant. Insulin resistance, they found, may actually play a role in leptin resistance in and of itself.

In a study performed in 1996, two groups of men were divided based on insulin resistance. Both groups of men were lean, with normal body fat indexes and body fat percentages of roughly 15%. The men were tested for their insulin sensitivity, which was determined based on an intravenous glucose tolerance test, and divided based on this finding. In men with increased insulin resistance, circulating levels of plasma leptin were found to be much higher, despite identical amounts of body fat. The researchers concluded that insulin resistance, even in normal-weight individuals, is associated with higher levels of plasma leptin. If elevated leptin levels lead to leptin resistance, this means that insulin resistance is directly affecting another hormonal pathway which encourages obesity.

Because of leptin resistance, Obese Americans live under constant brain signaling which causes the hypothalamus to believe they have minimal fat stores, even when 100 pounds overweight! If this is true, what would we expect to find when these individuals attempt to restrict their calories?

If the individual attempts to reduce calories from 3000 calories per day to 1500 calories per day, we would expect hormone signaling in the hypothalamus to induce extreme hunger and perseverating thoughts of food. Sound familiar? On most modern calorie-restriction diets, dieters think about food all day long and often go to bed hating their diets.

With leptin, this model finally makes sense. If modern Americans are resistant to leptin, the body thinks we are normal weight even when we are obese. If you lose 10 pounds from sheer willpower of exercise and diet, the body senses less leptin, because there are 10 pounds of fat missing from the previous metabolic inventory report. This decrease in leptin, in a brain that already has trouble seeing leptin, induces the mechanics of starvation and slowed metabolism despite regular feedings and maintenance of high amounts of body fat.

It Worked Until 1970

This situation sounds hopeless! But God did not design us this way. In the 1960s and before, the system worked. That is to say, before we began poisoning ourselves with the processed foods we have discussed in this book, the system worked almost flawlessly.

Picture you are a 1950's human. You have just eaten a rich and delicious dinner with friends on a special occasion; perhaps it was Susie's birthday. You went *way* over your supposed recommended calories. Susie likes to bake! After eating steak and mashed potatoes, you helped yourself to three pieces of birthday cake, lit a cigarette, and then drove home in your sky blue 1957 Chevy Bel Air.

In this 1950's scenario, your body responds by storing excess calories as fat, which then creates new leptin over the next 24-48 hours. This is leptin that your body has not seen before last night. The leptin signals to your hypothalamus that you have gained excess fat, so your hunger is severely decreased. Over the next 2-3 days, you eat very little, frowning at your plate as you have almost no appetite.

Simultaneously, your hypothalamus increases your metabolic rate through its effect on the thyroid. This causes your body to burn off some of this extra fat as energy. The hypothalamus then instructs your temperature set point to increase, so that excess fatty acids are burned as heat. Leptin, as it does in mice, then signals you to move more. So, at work that day, you fidget your knee and tap your foot. You click your pen and get up to go to the water cooler almost restlessly as your body attempts to burn off the excess calories.

When your fat stores return to normal levels, this leptin balance is restored. Your appetite returns, you stop tapping your foot, your body temperature returns to normal, and all is well in 1950s America.

Why Are We Leptin Resistant?

But this brings up the question: what is causing leptin resistance? So far, researchers have been unable to firmly expose the cause of leptin resistance. However, several theories exist. The one thing that researchers *have* been able to show is that insulin resistance and leptin resistance go hand in hand. If you are insulin resistant, you are, by definition, leptin-resistant also. Likewise, *fixing insulin resistance automatically fixes leptin resistance*.

It is possible that knowing this fact is enough for us at this point. Certainly, this will serve our purposes in this book. If we can fix our insulin resistance, we can restore our leptin sensitivity and get a double benefit. We will lower our obesity by lowering our insulin resistance, and moreover, we will return ourselves to the leptin sensitivity of the 1960s and before. But while we're on the subject, let's take a quick look at some proposed possibilities for leptin resistance.

Overstimulation vs. Inflammation

Theory One: Simply too much

The first theory is that we simply have too much circulating leptin because we are too fat. This creates, in much the same way as insulin resistance, a decreased sensitivity and decreased response to leptin. It is similar to a doorbell. If your doorbell rings once a month, you are very likely to answer it. If, however, you have a known prankster child in your neighborhood who rings your doorbell 4-5 times a day, you will very quickly begin to ignore that doorbell. The body is the same way. Overstimulation of a pathway of hormones leads to a decreased response. Your body simply cannot exhaust itself on all of your "crying wolf."

This argument makes some sense, but it seems somehow inadequate. It resembles the insulin resistance theories of scientists who argue "fat first, then insulin resistant." The problem with the argument of "fat first" is that it does not fully explain why we got fat in the first place. Put another way, why did the leptin hormone pathway work in the 1960s, but it does not work today? The second theory, however, may hold a more complete explanation.

Theory Two: Inflammation

The second theory posits that the inflammatory state of the body leads to certain receptors being activated in the hypothalamus, namely the TOR-4 Receptor (among others). These inflammatory pathways cause a cellular cascade (firing off of cell signals) which decreases leptin sensitivity.

Likewise, studies have shown that inflammation from the GI tract, when the "bad" bacteria are overgrown, lead to a buildup of something called lipopolysaccharide (or LPS), which causes a very strong inflammatory reaction in the body. This inflammatory signal has been shown to decrease both insulin sensitivity and leptin sensitivity in mice.

This theory is further substantiated by the fact that leptin-resistant mice seem to return to leptin sensitivity after fiber is introduced into their diets.

A Different Form of Diet

As I researched the biochemistry more and more, I wondered further, what would the human hormonal picture look like if you were able to **design a diet** that made you extremely **sensitive** to insulin and leptin. How would you feel if you dropped 10 or 20 lbs.? Would it feel like the calorie-restrictive "eat less exercise more diets" in which a person typically becomes fatigued, irritable, and hungry all the time?

Would hunger hormones rage and cause you to eat more to regain the weight? Would you want to stop moving and just lay in bed, while simultaneously feeling cold and grumpy? Would you get the same "weight-loss headache" that I had experienced throughout my yo-yo dieting?

As I created my own plan for eating to **maximize insulin and leptin sensitivity** and began to lose weight, the answer astounded me. Instead of feeling increasingly hungry as in previous diets, my hunger **decreased** as I lost weight. The more I lost, the more sensitive I became to both my circulating insulin and leptin. Leptin became more efficient at signaling my brain that I "had enough fat stores." I suffered no headaches, no irritability, no coldness. On the contrary, I felt jubilant. And almost every day I noticed my hunger was non-existent.

My body was becoming sensitive to leptin in ways it had never previously been. It was working like God intended! It was as if my hypothalamus was saying "Scott, even though you have lost 20 pounds, you are still very fat. Today we can just eat all of these stored calories. There is no need for you to have anything else to eat. Enjoy your day!" Never, in over a decade of attempting every diet known to man, had I felt anything like this.

As we move forward, we will look at the benefit of burning fat into ketones for fuel. In section three, we will put together the diet that is maximally designed to increase your leptin and insulin sensitivity, and cause weight loss like you have never experienced before.

Rule #5: I will strive to increase my sensitivity to Leptin. This will allow my body to "take inventory" of my fat stores, thereby decreasing my hunger and increasing my metabolism. To restore leptin sensitivity, I will first restore insulin sensitivity.

CHAPTER 9: **THE GLORY OF KETONES**

The History of Ketones

From 1878-1808, a US Army surgeon named Dr. Frederick Schwatka traveled 3,000 miles across the Canadian Arctic with two Inuit families, in search of the lost Franklin Expedition. The Franklin Expedition had gone looking for the Northwest Passage several years earlier but was never heard from again. During his time with the Inuit people, living in one of the harshest and coldest climates known to man, Dr. Schwatka ate a diet rich in meat and fat, with almost no carbohydrate. In his journal, he recorded something extraordinary.

"When first thrown wholly upon the diet of reindeer meat, it seems inadequate to properly nourish the system and there is an apparent weakness and inability to perform severe exertive, fatiguing journeys. But this soon passes away in the course of 2-3 weeks."

Eating only reindeer meat and fat, Dr. Schwatka experienced a fundamental transition in his body's metabolism of energy. Without glucose, his body, for the first time, was experiencing the dominance of the alternate fuel designed for him by God. He was experiencing Ketones. As his body was used to glucose as the primary fuel, it took roughly 2 weeks for his system to "reboot" and switch to ketones. But once he did so, he reported ***increased*** energy levels without the need for carbohydrates.

Thirty years later, Professor V Stefansson, a Harvard trained anthropologist, lived and traveled extensively with the Inuit people. From 1905 to 1917 Stefansson lived almost exclusively on Inuit food.

When he returned, he reported his diet and the health benefits which he enjoyed to the medical community of his time. But his writings were not well received. The medical community as a whole told him the diet he suggested, consisting of only animal fat and meat, was impossible. In effect, they called him a liar.

In 1928, to prove his truthfulness, Dr. Stefansson allowed himself to be held in Bellevue Mental Hospital in New York City, under constant guard, while he ate the same diet which he claimed to have eaten during his time with the Inuit people. True to his word, he stayed in his hospital room for over a year. During that time, his diet included virtually no carbohydrate. He ate 115 g of protein per day and greater than 200 grams of fat per day. Critics were certain he would die of scurvy within months. But Dr. Stefansson suffered no ill effects. Contrary to the belief of the time, Dr. Stefansson lost no muscle mass, maintained a healthy body weight, and did not develop scurvy or any other vitamin deficiency.

The medical community simply could not accept the fact that refined carbohydrates are unnecessary for the human diet. This is still true in modern nutrition. But human beings are not meant to live in a state of continual insulin dominance. By eating as modern American's do, with a diet continuously overloaded with refined carbohydrates and sugar, we have inhibited ourselves from ever enjoying the benefits of fat metabolism and ketones. And the benefits of ketone metabolism are many!

In the human system, neither dietary fat nor body fat can be turned into glucose. For this reason, when glucose is scarce, your body uses ketones, a chemical derived from fat breakdown, for energy in place of glucose. Throughout our history as human beings, prior to 1970, the hormonal picture of our bodies resembled a perfectly attuned pendulum, swinging from glucose metabolism to ketone metabolism. The pendulum, depending on the insulin to glucagon ratio, would alternate between these two vital fuels, allowing the human body to experience the benefit of both.

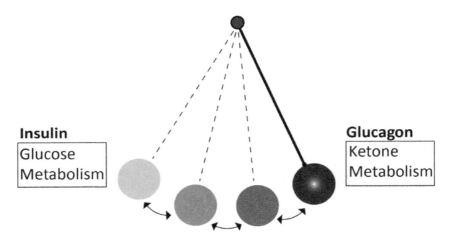

Insulin

Glucose Metabolism

Glucagon

Ketone Metabolism

Where our ancestors would switch to utilizing body fat for calorie needs within hours of their last meal, today we almost never switch into this mechanism. Our pendulum is stuck, fixed in the glucose-dominant state.

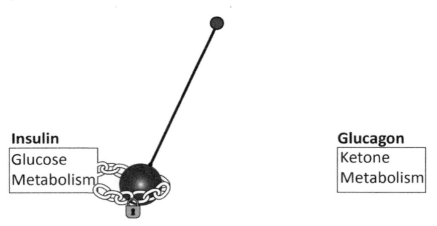

Insulin

Glucose Metabolism

Glucagon

Ketone Metabolism

To add insult to injury, the modern nutritionists insist we never miss a meal and eat as frequently as six times a day to maintain our metabolism! (Whatever the heck that means) So not only do we eat only foods which cause insulin resistance and high insulin levels, we make sure to eat them every 2-3 hours so that our body can *never* get a chance to switch back into fat metabolism. Our fat storage, for all intents and purposes, is eternally *locked*!

The Big Bad Ketone

Today the term "Ketone" or "Ketosis" is thrown around everywhere. Bloggers and Vloggers speak or write on the subject. People are warned about the harm of ketosis, with little regard for the truth of the matter. Even physicians ask ridiculous questions like: "is it safe to generate ketones for your body's calorie needs?" The fact that a physician could ask such a question is appalling. The human body is designed to run on ketones throughout our entire life. Some cultures, such as the Inuit, live almost **exclusively** on ketones. And guess what: they are very lean!

There is nothing more natural than using ketones for fuel. Ketones are the very way in which your body utilizes fat stores for energy. This is especially true in children. Have you ever wondered why children are so thin, and their parents are so fat? Throughout our life, the body switches to ketone metabolism more and more slowly. Since ketone generation equates to the burning of stored fat, the speed at which one enters ketosis is very important for weight loss. The graphic below illustrates the time necessary to begin generating ketones in modern America.

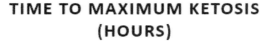

TIME TO MAXIMUM KETOSIS (HOURS)

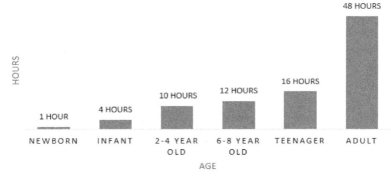

As you can see, a newborn baby can switch to the metabolism of fat for fuel in as little as 30-60 minutes after eating. As the study participant's age increased, this time became longer and longer. The modern American adult can take days to reach adequate ketone generation!

But is the modern American metabolism *meant* to take so much longer than the baby? My own theory is that this graph actually represents increasing insulin resistance, and not an age-based change in time to ketone metabolism. In other words, the adult on this graph has seen a lifetime of insulin-resistance causing foods. By the time the study is performed, he or she is in a metabolic state which takes 2-3 days to switch out of a high insulin: glucagon ratio and begin fully liberating fats from the tissue.

But what if our body was insulin sensitive? What if we quickly and efficiently switched between glucose and ketones as our main fuel? In such a scenario, it would be very difficult to maintain excess body weight. Moreover, as you will see, the body would gain significant other benefits.

Ketones, The Brain Super-Food

When it comes to utilizing ketones as our primary fuel, many unique advantages have been discovered. Think about it this way: if God invented two different fuels for your body to run on throughout your life, and we use only one of them (glucose) in modern America, is it possible that we are missing some wonderful advantages that the second fuel form may have for us? In other words, do ketones have effects that glucose does not, that we, as Americans, never see? In fact, they do.

Ketones have been shown to have protective effects for the brain. Studies have shown benefits to cognition, protection against Alzheimer's and dementia, epilepsy, and age-related mental deterioration.

In 1921 two incredibly important discoveries were made. First, Dr. Woodyatt noted that ketones appear in a normal human being after a period of fasting. Before this discovery, it was unclear what induced ketone creation. Meanwhile, Dr. Wilder of the Mayo

Clinic discovered that periods of fasting protected against seizures in patients with epilepsy. These doctors put two and two together. They theorized that the benefits of ketones generated during periods of fasting could be similarly induced if the body was limited to a low-carbohydrate diet. This diet could then be used to treat epilepsy.

Wilder proposed a manner of eating, which he termed a "Ketogenic Diet," to be tried in a series of patients with epilepsy. His hope was that the diet would be as effective as fasting and could be maintained for a much longer period of time. After all, starving the epilepsy patients would not solve the problem. His dietary recommendations were for 1 gram of protein per kilogram of weight, less than 10-15 grams of carbohydrate per day, and the remainder of calories to be eaten as fat.

In subjects who adhered to his diet, 52% had complete remission of their seizures, and an additional 27% had significant improvement in the number and intensity of seizures. Subsequent to this result, the ketogenic diet appeared in every comprehensive neurology textbook on epilepsy between 1941 and 1980.

In a 2001 study, this effect was demonstrated again. Epileptic children begun on a ketogenic (high fat low carbohydrate) diet for more than 1-year experienced similar results. Nearly half of the study participants experienced a greater than 90% remission of all seizure activity. In many children, the diet allowed a decrease or discontinuation of medication without a relapse into seizures.

Dr. Peterman of the Mayo clinic, studying the same effect, noted that the ketogenic diet also led to improvements in behavior and cognitive function in the participants.

Beyond protection against seizures, many individuals feel "clearer" during times of ketone metabolism. The brain has long been accustomed to utilizing ketones for energy, and some studies suggest that it prefers a 33/67 ketone to glucose mix, rather than the 100% pure glucose on which it usually subsides in general American culture.

A 2004 study found that Alzheimer's patients treated with a ketogenic diet had increased memory and cognitive ability assessed with the Alzheimer's Disease Assessment Scale. This increase in memory correlated precisely with serum ketone levels. In other words, the more ketones the patient generated, the better their memory.

In 2018 a study was performed to evaluate the effects of a ketogenic diet on children suffering from autism. Fifteen children, aged from 2 to 17 years, were observed for 3-6 months. Of these children, all experienced significant improvement in cognitive testing. Researchers also noted improvements in imitation, body use, and fear or nervousness after 3 months.

As I personally have switched to elevated ketone generation through manipulation of my insulin: glucagon ratio, my own clarity has increased dramatically. My energy levels are similarly elevated.

The Anti-inflammatory and Anti-Oxidant Ketone

Beyond the protection of our brain-health, ketones potently increase your body's own natural anti-oxidants. Modern America is obsessed with foods "rich in anti-oxidants," but yet we neglect the primary anti-oxidant which God created for your system! In a study looking at human genes which produce natural anti-oxidants, the genetic sequence which creates these potent chemicals were found to be "switched-on" by increased ketone levels.

This means your body has "sleeper genes," waiting for the signal of high ketone levels to activate them. These genes then produce potent anti-oxidants which search for harmful free radicals within the body. "Free Radicals" are chemical molecules which like to "oxidize" or bind to almost anything, including DNA, where they have been shown to cause mutations and possibly lead to cancer.

The fear of free radicals is why so many foods today boast "Natural Anti-oxidants." But what if the body has its own incredible mechanisms of fighting free radicals, which we never activate because we never allow ourselves to use ketones as fuel?

Beyond anti-oxidant production, Ketones have been shown to be highly anti-inflammatory. We discussed in our section on leptin that both insulin and leptin resistance have been linked to inflammation. Perhaps our inflammatory states in modern America are due to the fact that we almost never metabolize ketones for fuel?

In 2008, a study was performed comparing the effects of a low-fat diet versus a very low carbohydrate diet on inflammation. Researchers found an overall anti-inflammatory effect associated with a very low carbohydrate diet, which resulted in decreases in 7 out of the 7 inflammatory markers tested. Other studies have corroborated this finding, linking ketones to decreased whole-body inflammation.

In the model of the pendulum, our body is meant to utilize insulin and glucose, then revert to glucagon and ketone metabolism, which reduces inflammation, and increases insulin sensitivity. The one side of the pendulum protects the other side of the pendulum. But we don't allow it to do so!

Starving Cancer

Amazing new research being done at Duke University, and elsewhere, is exploring the possibility that ketone metabolism may protect against cancer. In the last 100 years, cancer rates have increased dramatically. The cause is not well understood.

However, in the 1920s, Nobel laureate Otto Warburg found that cancer cells thrive on the breakdown of glucose. Could this be linked to our increasing cancer rates? Through a process called "Anaerobic metabolism," cancer cells utilize glucose for energy in the absence of oxygen.

Cancer cells prefer this type of metabolism, even when oxygen is abundant. Cancer, too aggressive to wait for sufficient oxygen in order to grow, simply breaks down glucose without it. By forgoing oxygen, the cancer is able to grow as large as it wants, without worrying about sufficient oxygen levels.

However, fatty acid metabolism *requires* oxygen. Hence cancer cells cannot utilize fatty acids to grow. In light of this, scientists have theorized that cancer's preference for glucose may be the greatest possible weakness of this deadly disease. Researchers theorize that a diet low in glucose and rich in ketone metabolism may likewise stop cancer before it starts.

In 2017 the Journal of Medical Oncology published a review of all known literature supporting the assertion that ketogenic diets may protect against cancer. The review evaluated 29 animal studies and 24 human studies. The review found that 72% of the animal studies yielded significant evidence for an anti-tumor effect of ketogenic diets. Because no strong human trials have yet been done, the review limited human evidence to anecdotal case reports throughout history. However, the case reports represent very promising patient stories.

In 1922, Braunstein noted that glucose disappeared from the urine of diabetic patients after a cancer diagnosis. The finding suggested that glucose is "stolen away" by the cancer cells, and is necessary for cancer growth.

In 1962, the New York Department of Mental Hygiene published a case report about two women suffering from cancer. The women's cancers, one skin cancer, and the other cervical cancer were both advanced, and visible on external examination of the body. Both patients, as fate would have it, also happened to be undergoing psychiatric therapy. This therapy consisted of daily medically-induced hypoglycemia (low blood sugar). After 2 months of this therapy, both cancers became undetectable. It was proposed that the hypoglycemia starved cancer cells of glucose, leading to their elimination.

In 1995, two pediatric patients suffering from astrocytoma (brain cancer) were fed a ketogenic diet for 8 weeks. During this time their PET-CT (head scans) showed promising improvements with decreased glucose uptake within their tumor sites. Of the two patients, one continued on the diet and remained disease-free.

Rigorous randomized studies evaluating the effects of

ketogenic diets on cancer are currently being performed at Duke University, Tel Aviv Sourasky Medical Center, and St. Joseph's Hospital and Medical Center of Phoenix, AZ. As time goes by, it is likely more and more evidence will corroborate the case reports of the past.

Though the research is not complete, we may perform a simple, common-sense exercise to evaluate the postulated theory. If a diet rich in ketones protects against cancer, then we would expect to see a glucose-rich environment inducing higher cancer rates. The person in whom we would expect to see the highest cancer rates, therefore, would be an untreated type 2 diabetic, with blood glucose levels constantly elevated. Do we see an increased risk of cancer in uncontrolled type 2 diabetes? Yes, we do. The rates of cancer with poor blood glucose control (an HA1C > 6.5) increase 400%, with greater increases in cancer risk correlating to higher levels of glucose.

The Wasted Ketone

Beyond brain protection and postulated cancer protection, ketones have effects on our weight control which are absolutely amazing, and most relevant to our study on weight loss. Chief among these benefits is the ability for ketones to be "wasted" by the body. As Ketones circulate in your bloodstream, some ketone bodies degrade into acetone.

Acetone is highly evaporative. In our modern world, acetone is often used to remove nail polish and paint. As anyone who has ever worked with acetone can tell you, if you leave the cap off the bottle, it evaporates very quickly. It evaporates so quickly, in fact, that a person in ketosis often breathe and urinates off as many as 20 calories every hour.

That's right! When you are in a state of ketone generation, your body is **breathing off fat** from your body. Fat is literally evaporating off of your buttocks, belly, and hips into the air around you. I don't know about you, but that is my kind of weight loss!

This is well known in medicine. Diabetics can enter a state

called ketoacidosis. This is a pathologic state, unknown to healthy bodies, in which there is zero insulin, and high levels of glucagon. This leads to insanely high levels of fat breakdown in the body, as well as supranormal levels of both ketones and acetone in the bloodstream. This leads to acidic blood or "Keto-acidosis."

In medical school, one of the ways physicians are taught to detect ketoacidosis is by the smell of the patient. There is often a musky or fruity smell, which is detected when the physician smells the patient's breath. This musky-fruity smell is acetone! While this is very dangerous for a type 1 diabetic such as myself, for a non-diabetic, ketone levels never climb this high, and are *not dangerous*. Expelling acetone in the breath is, therefore, something to be celebrated.

Acetone can also be wasted through the urine. A common way to detect the metabolic state of ketosis is urine testing. Often a color-changing urine dipstick is used to test for the presence of ketones in the urine. When present, ketones turn the color of the dipstick from light tan to deep purple.

As a physician who has tested thousands of urine samples in the ER, I can tell you *definitively* that the modern American has very little to *no* ketone presence in their urine! Indeed, almost no person whose urine sample I have tested has any baseline ketosis. This means that almost none of my patients are burning *any* fat. Conversely, my own urine tests "high" for ketones at any time during the day, 24/7, even after meals. The only difference is the manipulation of my hormones through diet. This is staggering!

If we can enter a state where we create ketones from our fat, our body will literally urinate our buttocks, hips, and flabby bellies into the toilet for us. At the same time, it will breathe and sweat them away. Do you still think God had no mechanism for our body to lose weight? Or did we just miss part of the equation?

The Brown Fat Machine

But wait, there's more! In the body, there are two types of fat cells. These are known as "White Fat" and "Brown Fat" cells. The difference is microscopic but incredibly important. In White Fat, levels of mitochondria are very low, leading to a "white" appearance under the microscope. Brown Fat, on the other hand, has very high levels of mitochondria, and so appears "brown" under the microscope.

Brown Fat, rich in mitochondria, is a type of fat cell meant to burn or waste fatty acids for heat generation. This fat exists for two purposes. The first is to keep you warm, but the second is to waste excess calories in times of overfeeding, thereby maintaining your healthy weight. Mitochondria are the crucial difference. Mitochondria are the organelle (cellular organ) in which all fatty acids are metabolized for fuel or heat. And the brown fat is brimming with them to the point of changing the basic color of the cell!

Studies have been done which show that baby fat is mostly brown fat. It has been theorized that this is why babies do not shiver when taken into a cold environment, and likewise why their transition to ketone metabolism is so rapid. Their cute roly-poly arms and legs are teeming with brown fat, ready to generate heat at a moment's notice from the fatty acids they have ingested from breast milk.

White fat, on the other hand, has only one purpose. White fat's single function is to store body fat. With very little mitochondria, white fat is very poor at metabolizing fatty acids for heat or energy. It is white fat, and not brown, which increases when a person becomes obese. Their body becomes rich in stores of white fat on their buttocks, thighs, and abdomen. It is white fat which all of us are eager to shed!

Recent studies have shown something mind-boggling. In rats, diets rich in ketones have led to the conversion of white fat into brown fat. Let me restate that! Ketones cause the conversion of harmful white storage fat into metabolism-boosting brown fat! This brown fat then aids in the wasting of excess pounds throughout the body by burning excess fat for heat! We would, therefore, expect someone with increased amounts of brown fat to have a higher baseline metabolism, and to be much more resistant to weight gain.

A 2014 study performed on rats showed that the volume of space occupied by the mitochondria in brown fat increased by a whopping 60% after a one-month ketogenic diet. Likewise, the enzymes associated with fat metabolism increased by 300%!

How Do We Change Our Hormonal Picture?

As you can see, the benefits of ketone metabolism are amazing. Up to this point in our study on weight maintenance, we have discussed the changes to our diet which have led to insulin resistance, and subsequently, how those changes influence our body's hormones.

In the next section, we will talk about the simple changes a person can make to the way they live and eat, which will heal their insulin resistance and leptin resistance. This hormonal healing will lead you, as it did with me, to increased glucose control, round-the-clock ketone generation, and potent weight loss. We will return you to the system which God designed for you: a system in which it is *impossible to become obese*.

Rule #6: I will strive to make ketones my predominant body-fuel. I will not allow glucose and insulin to dominate my metabolism.

Section IV

Healing Our Insulin Resistance

CHAPTER 10: **TIME RESTRICTED FEEDING AND FASTING**

Fixing Our Insulin Resistance

Throughout the first and second sections of this book, we have looked at the changes to the American diet since the 1950s, as well as the hormonal problems these changes cause within our bodies. It is time, now, to explore how a modern American can undo these changes and revert the damage of insulin and leptin resistance.

The goal, then, is to give the body breaks from the glucose-full, insulin-elevated, non-ketone state in which nearly all Americans reside. We want to give our body periods of rest, during which the normal mechanisms of weight loss can begin to kick in. To undo all this damage, we will look at the two most important aspects of insulin sensitivity: when to eat, and what to eat.

What may surprise you, as it surprised me, is that modern research shows that *when* we eat is *far* more important than *what* we eat. In modern America, nutritionists and dieticians teach that we must eat every 2-3 hours to maintain our metabolism and achieve optimal weight loss. This is based on zero definitive scientific evidence, yet it is taught as gospel truth. Trusting their educators, modern Americans believe this advice. The American dieter, therefore, eats breakfast, mid-morning snack, lunch, mid-afternoon snack, dinner, and before-bed snack at reduced calorie levels, all in an effort to lose weight. This is mind-boggling; The modern American eats *all day* to lose weight! It seems ridiculous. But as a physician, I was susceptible to this bad advice too. I followed and tried the "eat small meals all day" plan. Did I lose weight? Not a pound.

The hormonal result of this style of eating is a never-ending cycle of insulin spikes throughout the hours of the day. After each insulin spike, the pendulum of ketone metabolism is fixed firmly in the "off position," and glucose remains the dominant fuel.

As you consider the standard "low calorie" snacks which people eat, you will notice something: they are all high sugar, high carbohydrate products. The modern American, adhering to modern dietary advice, starts off with highly refined oatmeal for breakfast (insulin spike), followed by a sugary yogurt for mid-morning snack (insulin spike). He or she then eats a sandwich with low-fat mayonnaise for lunch (insulin spike), followed by rice cakes for mid-afternoon snack (insulin spike). For dinner, he or she eats a calorie-reduced portion of meat and rice (insulin spike), followed by a late-night snack of non-fat frozen yogurt (insulin spike). The result is a graph of insulin throughout the day which looks like this:

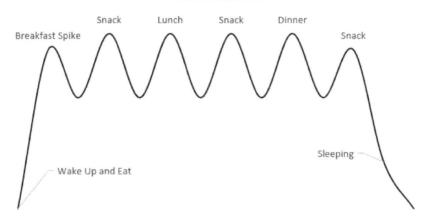

Insulin Levels

Effectively, this modern American has just maintained insulin at near-peak levels the *entire* day. The peaked insulin signals the body to maintain fat stores at all costs, to avoid the burning of fat into ketones, and to attempt to gain weight! Glucagon is held at low levels resulting in a high insulin: glucagon ratio.

The failure of this type of diet has been extensively studied. What is interesting is that no matter how much a person reduces their calories (1500, 1200, 900), insulin still instructs the body "Do Not Burn Fat." It is that simple. But if the body is receiving fewer calories, and has been told not to burn its reserve fuel (fat), what answer does it have left? The only answer the body has is to reduce total calorie expenditure, which means *lowering metabolism*.

Fasting for Health

If eating six small meals throughout the day (sometimes called grazing) is not the answer, then what is? In our effort to undo insulin resistance, we must find the most effective way to create insulin sensitivity throughout the day, while minimizing insulin resistance when we eat. Humans have known how to do this throughout all of human history. But somehow, we have forgotten. The answer, simply put, is fasting.

Throughout history, every major culture and religion has fasted. Christians, Muslims, Jews, and Hindus (as well as many other faiths) all have periods of fasting. Spiritual reasons aside, fasting has also been done for the purposes of beating disease, general physical health, mental clarity, increased energy levels, and of course, weight loss. Throughout human history, fasting was never seen as harmful; rather, it was seen as miraculous for its benefits on health. *Fasting is not starvation*. Fasting is the purposeful abstaining from food for a determined period of time. And the greats throughout history knew that it worked.

Hippocrates, widely acknowledged as the father of modern medicine, recommended eating "only once a day" to promote health. Plutarch, an ancient Greek writer, philosopher, and historian, stated:

"instead of using medicine, better fast today." Plato and Aristotle, titans of philosophy and science, also strongly supported fasting. Plato stated, "I fast for greater physical and mental efficiency."

In the early 1500s, the European physician Paracelsus, the founder of the discipline of toxicology (the study of toxins and poisons on the human body) stated that fasting was "the greatest remedy" and the body's "physician within." Benjamin Franklin, one of America's founding fathers, wrote, "The best of all medicines is resting and fasting." Even Mark Twain knew this. Twain wrote, "A little starvation can really do more for the average sick man than can the best medicines and the best doctors."

I know what you are thinking. "Starvation? That's the answer?!?" Not at all! This has nothing to do with starvation. Rather, we are talking about giving our body *times each day* in which we *do not eat*, and a reciprocal time each day in which we *do* eat. Doing so allows the pendulum of glucose to ketone metabolism to swing naturally and healthfully back and forth, the way it was intended.

Think about it this way. Everyone accepts that sleep is necessary. It is taught that during sleep, we regenerate tissue, repair damage from the day, and process the day's information in the form of dreams. Since we have two phases of human existence (awake and asleep), and both perform critical functions for our health, is it unreasonable to suggest that the human body has two critical metabolic states (fed and unfed) which perform equally critical tasks?

What studies suggest is that human beings need periods without food to begin ketone and fat metabolism, and to promote amazing benefits for the body. This is in stark contrast to the modern idea that we must eat every 2-3 hours to lose weight. God designed your body so that the periods without food reset your internal machinery. During times of fasting, your body resets its insulin sensitivity and blooms into the myriad of benefits seen from ketone metabolism. Mercifully, God made it so this time without food does not have to be very long at all.

In modern studies, beginning with the studies on fasting performed by famed endocrinologist George Cahill in 1970, we have found that the body usually begins depleting a great part of the glycogen (glucose stores), at around hour 9 after eating. The body then begins to pull fat from your fat stores and begins using ketones for fuel.

Simultaneously, insulin levels begin to drop after you finish eating, reaching their lowest point after this 9-hour marker. In tandem with falling insulin, glucagon begins to rise until peaking somewhere around hour 8.

After only 9 hours of fasting, we enter into a healthy insulin: glucagon ratio. Ketones begin to emerge from the liver. Fat cells begin to spill fatty acids into the bloodstream and your excess body fat begins to shrink. Mitochondria activate to burn fat as heat and energy. Inflammation reduces. The clouds clear, the sun comes out, and the body enters into a repair and maintenance phase.

Lower insulin levels begin the process of healing our insulin resistance, increasing both our insulin and leptin sensitivity. After only 9 hours without food, our body begins the process of undoing our abysmal food choices. But do we let it? Sleep is the most natural phase of fasting for most modern human beings. During sleep, you eat no calories. Yet even a modern dietician would not advise you to rise every 2 hours from sleep in order to eat and "keep your metabolism up."

Still, most Americans eat until the time they go to bed, and then again immediately after they wake up in the morning. As Americans sleep, on average, 6.8 hours per night, this means the only rest from insulin that we give our body is frighteningly short! This 6.8-hour window of fasting falls 2 hours short of the 9-hour mark when our body would begin to utilize fat stores for energy.

How many hours do Americans eat?

Scientists at USC, leading researchers in circadian rhythm and mammalian sleep, did a study in 2015 to assess how many hours of the day the average American eats. The study was ingenious, and the findings were stunning.

In the experiment, the researchers first asked participants to estimate how many hours they eat in a day. What would your answer be when asked such a question? Most of the study participants answered, "roughly 12 to 13 hours". The participants estimated eating from 8 AM, until roughly 8 or 9 pm.

The participants were then asked to take photos of their food in an app designed for the study. Researchers could then review the photos generated from the app and map out the exact times the person ate.

What the study found surprised both the researchers as well as the participants. On average, Americans ate 15 hours per day. The average food intake began at 7:30 AM with coffee, creamed and sugared, as well as a sugary breakfast food. Typically, this was cereal or some other product rich in refined carbohydrates. The participants were then noted to eat often throughout the entire day, snacking between meals and well into the late evening. They often recorded their last food intake as late as 11 PM or Midnight. For me, this was very familiar. I often found myself snacking while watching TV with my wife late at night. Stopping at 11 pm, I would then sleep until about 7 AM when I awoke for work. Even as a diabetic, my first meal was carbohydrate-rich toast, and a nice big shot of insulin!

Let's stop and think about 15 hours of eating in the context of ketone creation: 24 hours – 15 hours of eating = 9 hours of fasting. As Ketone production kicks off after 9 hours of fasting, modern Americans are eating just long enough to ***never*** enter the time of ketone production. Let me say this again as it is perhaps the most important thing you will ever hear regarding weight loss! In America, we ***never*** let our body create ketones. After eating for 15 hours, we sleep for 8 or 9 hours, then repeat the process, never letting our glycogen deplete, never letting our system switch to ketones for fuel, and never letting our insulin: glucagon ratio transition to healthy levels. In the morning, we eat a carbohydrate-rich food, stimulating insulin production. We then repeat the cycle every day, week in, week out. We have no rest from insulin, the hormone which instructs our body to store fat.

But it was not always so. In the time before electricity, historians have shown that we often went to bed not long after nightfall. As the sun went down, without electric lights, we began to have natural circadian sleepiness. Candles allowed us to stay awake a bit longer and read. Fireplaces helped us chat and finish our supper, but in the end, the brain hormones inducing sleep won, and we went to bed. Even if this only resulted in the cessation of eating 4 hours earlier, which it most certainly did, this meant that every day we had 4 hours of ketone metabolism which we have lost today.

Even in times of electricity, fasting windows were historically longer. In the 1950s, it was far more common to eat breakfast, lunch, and finally a 6:30 pm dinner. In my interviews with people who lived through the 1950s and 1960s, almost all stated the same thing: "We ate three meals, barely snacked, and stopped at about 6:30 pm." If this is true, this would suggest the fasting interval in the 1950s and 1960s was roughly the same as that of the pre-electricity era and would represent an eating window of 11 hours a day (depending on the timing of breakfast). This would result in 3-5 hours of ketone use, as well as decreased insulin level, decreased insulin resistance, and decreased leptin resistance.

In my interviews, people who recall this era also pointed out that some of the things we do in today's world would never be accepted. There were food taboos. One individual put it to me this way, "Today you see a guy walking down the street eating a taco, or eating at his desk while at work. That just didn't happen". He went on to explain, "After dinner, I would never have been allowed a snack. It was dinner and done at my house." I'll let you speak to the individuals in your own life who may remember whether this is true or not, but still, it is a fascinating insight.

Time-Restricted Feeding and the Benefits of Fasting

Dr. Satchin Panda, the leading researcher in circadian rhythm, is also the world's expert on Time-Restricted Feeding. Time-Restricted Feeding refers to eating every day within a certain time interval. Dr. Panda decided to use the term "time-restricted feeding" because he found that the term "fasting" was often connected with the idea of calorie restriction. But Dr. Panda's work *does not include calorie restriction*.

Dr. Panda and his team, while studying mice, began to experiment with the timing of their feeding. His results have provided some of the most fascinating insights into the benefits of longer fasting windows (time without food) that have ever been recorded.

Dr. Panda took two groups of *genetically identical* mice and fed them in two different ways. The first group he allowed to graze all day. The second group of mice was allowed to eat during a 9-hour feeding window. The other 15 hours were spent fasting. Both groups ate the same number of calories and the exact same type of food. Let me restate this, as we have been so trained on the importance of calories: both groups ate the *same number of calories* and the *same food*. The results were astounding.

First, and perhaps most relevant to this book, the group fed in the 9-hour window reduced their body fat by 70%. That's right, a 70% reduction in body fat by simply changing *when* the mice ate. Holy Cow! This would be the equivalent of two modern Americans both eating 15 candy bars per day as their only food. If one person ate these candy bars throughout the entire day, while the other ate them in a specific time window, one person would lose weight, while the other would not! The fasted mice were likewise noted to have dramatically improved tolerance to glucose, with lower overall insulin levels and significantly lower insulin resistance.

Secondly, the fasted mice lowered their inflammatory markers. Inflammation decreased across every major inflammatory marker tested. This corroborates our study on the effects of ketones as highly anti-inflammatory. As noted earlier in this book, decreased inflammation leads to increased insulin sensitivity and leptin sensitivity, thereby lowering the hormones in your body which signal fat storage. This, no doubt, helped the 70% reduction in fat mass seen in the mice.

Thirdly, and perhaps most surprisingly, the fasted mice had a nearly 20% increase in muscle tone. Yes, you read that right. The fasted mice had 20% more lean muscle after eating during a specific time window. So much for the bodybuilders who think they must eat all day to gain muscle!

Next, the fasted mice increased their mitochondrial volume. Remember when we discussed brown fat? Brown fat cells are the beneficial fat cells. They burn fat for heat, rather than storing it on your thighs. The fasted mice had an increase in both the number and size of their mitochondria, indicating white fat was actively being converted to brown fat. This makes sense when considered! If your body needs to run on fat during regular fasting windows, it makes sense for your body to ramp up and increase the organelles which do the job. That is exactly what we see in these mice. This means at all times, whether feeding or not feeding, these mice became better at burning excess body fat.

Lastly, the researchers noted an increase in autophagy and auto repair. Autophagy is the process by which the body "cleans up" old cells. In the body, as a cell stops functioning at peak performance, it is discarded and then cleared away by the body's natural systems. Autophagy, Latin for "self-eat," is the natural process by which this occurs. The body's immune cells "eat" the old cells, keeping your system running at its maximum potential, without the clutter of dying and dysfunctional cells in the way.

In medicine, we have termed these worn-out, discarded cells "senescent" cells. They are also sometimes referred to as "zombie" cells because they are not quite dead and not quite alive. Many modern scientists believe the key to longevity lies in understanding the role of these zombie cells. Recently, scientists have discovered that when the body persists in a high insulin state, autophagy, much like fat burning, is inhibited. For this reason, old cells seem to stack up. During ketone metabolism, the inhibition on this process is removed, and the body begins to *clean house*.

As "zombie" cells increase inflammation, they also increase insulin resistance. As they stack up further and further in a person who never utilizes ketones, insulin resistance from inflammation worsens. This leads to another cycle of insulin resistance, higher insulin levels, and further inhibition of autophagy.

Similarly, it has been shown that during the hours of ketone metabolism and fasting, the body begins to repair our DNA. The genes which are responsible for correcting any mutations in DNA, which can lead to cancer, are activated during times of elevated glucagon and ketone metabolism. So not only does a rest from eating activate "house-cleaning" of old and dysfunctional cells, but it increases the "repair mode" of DNA proofreading.

Pretend your body is a city. When you are in a high glucose and insulin state, the city planning board is in a full grow, grow, grow mode. The city planners forgo all repair of highways, bridges, and old buildings, favoring instead to dispatch the building crews of the city to build *new* highways, *new* bridges, and *new* buildings. Conversely, when you are in a low glucose, low insulin state, the city board shifts its focus. It is no longer important to build new highways, bridges, or buildings; rather, the city board places all of its focus on repairing older structures. It even goes back over all the old blueprints and city-planning schematics to check for errors.

In much the same way, when you are in a high insulin and glucose state, your body increases fat cell size and is signaled only to worry about growth. It even declines to perform the basic function of clearing out old, useless cells. During a ketone state, induced by fasting, your body begins to check and recheck its work. Old cells are cleared away, DNA is repaired, and the system is streamlined. These findings indicate that the body is *meant to fast*, and repair, daily. In America, is it any wonder our cancer rates, as well as our obesity, are through the roof? Is it likewise any wonder that obesity itself leads to higher cancer rates? The thing which makes us obese also stops us from auto-repairing our bodies!

Lastly, the fasted mice were found to have higher coordination, improved heart function, and improved endurance. All good things! Indeed, there were no negative effects whatsoever.

Benefits of a 12 Hour Fast

From the data, it is clear that Americans need longer periods between eating. Great. But how long? On this point, there is much contention. In Dr. Panda's study, after asking his participants to send in pictures of their food, timestamped to provide information on **when** they ate, Dr. Panda asked willing participants to go further. He asked them to narrow their feeding window to 11 hours, leaving another 13 hours for fasting.

This is a very gentle request. Could you lessen the hours in which you eat down to 11 hours? For example, 10 am to 9 pm. Of course, you could! Among participants, the average weight loss over 16 weeks was 7.2 pounds (3.27 kg). This weight was lost **without changing the type or amount** of food eaten or increasing exercise. Some participants saw significantly more weight loss, all for doing nothing more than allowing their body a **slightly** longer rest between eating. If we get this benefit simply from narrowing our eating window to 11 hours, what would happen if we narrowed our eating window further? This is exactly what I sought to find out.

The Ideal Eating Window

Many types of fasting or "time-restricted feeding" diets exist today. The "5/2 Diet" advocates a diet of eating normally for 5 days and fasting for 2 days each week. Alternative day fasting, similarly, recommends fasting every other day. The 16/8 diet recommends eating for 8 hours and fasting for 16 hours at least 5 days per week, with two days of allowed "all day eating." The OMAD diet (One Meal A Day) advocates eating all of your daily calories within one, usually half-hour, meal per day. The Warrior diet recommends one large meal per day, with light snacking allowed in the form of raw vegetables and certain fruits.

In an effort to test all of these methods, I performed each type of fasting for two weeks. My goal was to note differences in ketone metabolism and weight loss between the many variations. Each style of fasting has advantages, but also limitations.

For example, in both the 5/2 and Alternating Day form of fasting, which advocate whole days of fasting interspersed between days of normal eating, I found that the day after a fast my hunger was increased, I was slightly irritable, and I suffered from a slight headache. This was less than ideal.

Both the 5/2 and Alternate Day fasting allow you to eat as many as 500 calories on your "fast day." However, it is not dictated that these 500 calories be eaten in any certain time-window. As my goal was to obtain both weight loss and the benefits which Dr. Panda showed in his time-restricted mice, I have concerns about any diet which asks me to simply calorie restrict on certain days. My goal is not calorie restriction, as we have discussed many times in this book, but rather hormonal rebalancing. Diets which do not mandate a time window for eating, theoretically, would allow a person to eat small carbohydrate calorie loads throughout their fast day, effectively keeping their insulin high on the "fast day," and leading to continued insulin resistance. During these diets, I found my ketone generation to be stunted based on *when* I ate, and weight loss was, as expected, underwhelming.

The OMAD diet is very effective for ketone generation and weight loss. One meal a day, however, was too long for me to wait before eating. I would find myself watching the clock, wishing the magical meal of the day would arrive. I have no intention of living this way. Weight loss and ketone generation were magnificent while eating one meal a day. However, as a lifestyle choice, it was not for me.

Conversely, eating small amounts of vegetables throughout the day while eating one large meal at 7 pm, similar to the Warrior

Diet, required me to take small doses of insulin to keep my blood glucose in normal limits. As insulin is the weight gain hormone, this was less than ideal. This led to slowed weight loss and decreased ketone generation.

In general, I very much liked the 16 and 8 style of eating (16 hours fasting and 8 hours of eating). With the 16/8 I found ketone generation to be decent and had no ill effects of irritability, or lifestyle impairment. I lost weight reliably, and insulin demands decreased.

However, over time, my hunger consistently decreased. Each day, listening to my body's natural hunger, I found I wanted to eat in a smaller and smaller time window. The sweet spot on which I eventually settled, is an eating window of 4-5 hours. When eating 4-5 hours per day, I found I had no trouble throughout the morning waiting for lunch at 3 pm. Similarly, I was then able to eat a beautiful dinner at 7 or 8 pm, and not perseverate on food for the rest of the evening. Superior to the 16/8, my urine and blood ketone levels remained elevated for roughly 15 hours of the day, indicating a strong maintenance of a high glucagon, low insulin state. Similarly, my insulin needs declined most steadily and most impressively when utilizing a 4-5 hour eating window.

Therefore, to my patients, I strongly recommend a 20:4 (or 19:5) fasting to eating window. This is based on how well I lost weight, my ketone levels generated, my decrease in insulin requirement, and how others I have coached have performed. *Without exception, my most effective weight loss was done through an eating window of 4-5 hours per day, with a resulting fast of 19-20 hours.*

During my weight loss of 116 pounds, I ate from 4 pm to 8 pm. The remaining hours I drank coffee, water, and even diet soda (more on artificial sweeteners later). During fasting, my only intention was to avoid anything which may require the use of insulin. As such, these hours were calorie-free, as all macronutrients require at least some insulin, with carbohydrates requiring the most. With this eating window, and with the diet alterations we will discuss in the next chapter, I lost as many as 8 lbs. in a single week, with an average loss of 5.5 lbs per week. What's more, this was *without any type of exercise*. That's right. I sat on my large rear-end, without a single drop of sweat from exercise, and lost almost 6 lbs every week, simply by changing my eating window and diet.

With a 4-5 hour eating window, I suffered no irritability, no headache, and no feelings of starvation. In truth, I felt quite contented. Today, it is only if I eat outside of this normal window that I feel slightly nauseated or sick. Hunger levels throughout my fasting period are non-existent. Imagine if someone woke you up from deep sleep at 3 am and tried to force-feed you a snack. Would you be in the mood to eat? Or would you say "leave me alone, I'm sleeping!". After your body becomes accustomed to eating during certain hours of the day, you naturally feel this same reaction when offered food outside of your designated eating time.

How Hard Will This Be?

Time-restricted eating is the simplest and most effective thing you could start today for weight loss and insulin sensitivity, and once you get started, it is the easiest thing in the world! Many of those I have coached in weight loss were stuck, simply plateaued in their insulin resistance and leptin resistance, eating 1200 calories a day yet losing no weight, or worse, gaining it back. The simple recommendation to eat in a 4-hour window, rather than throughout the day, led one of my participants to lose 12 pounds in two weeks after being stuck at her same weight for 3 months!

The rest had similar results. The body is very adaptable. What we find in people who are new to restricted eating windows is that, for about three days, the body has predictable insulin spikes throughout the day. This has been trained over years of eating. You have taught your body when you normally eat, and for this reason, your body anticipates you, like an alarm clock, by sending out insulin *before* you eat. In this way, your hunger is already decided by a previous version of yourself. And so, fasting throughout the early day can be tough for the first three days.

After about three days of fasting throughout the early day, however, your body decides to stop sending out these pulses of insulin and ghrelin (the hunger hormone), and you feel naturally "unhungry" until you get to your determined eating window. Throughout all of the many individuals who I have coached, all tell me the same thing: "For about three days I was hungry in the morning. Then suddenly, I felt great and had no trouble lasting until my eating window". I experienced this, and so will you.

When we eat for a 4-5-hour window, our body will exist in a ketone-generating state for at least 10 hours each day. By modifying the diet which we will discuss in the next chapter, we can further enhance that window, as I did, to roughly 22 hours. But at the minimum, you will have 10 hours of pure fat burning, which God designed into the natural program of how our bodies are supposed to work. It is only in this modern generation that we do not give our bodies the chance to enter this state. During this time of ketone generation, you will have the benefit of burning away your excess body fat, increasing insulin sensitivity, and promoting muscle growth. Your metabolic rate will go up; white fat will convert to brown fat, and rather than plateauing your weight loss, you will see it ramp up every week.

First Steps:

As you begin to restrict your own eating window, it is perfectly acceptable to work up to a 4-hour window. If you prefer, begin with a 10-12-hour window, the next day, take it to 9, then 8, and so on over a week or so. If you are not feeling hungry as your insulin levels re-arrange themselves, push it further. Your goal is to choose a 4-5 hours window (my own personal window is 4 pm to 8 pm) and eat all of your calories during that time. During the rest of the day drink black coffee, tea, or water. Your only goal during the period of fasting is to avoid surges of insulin, and these will not occur if you avoid foods with calories.

During my own personal fasting, I drink diet soda. The decision to do the same is up to you. In Chapter 14 of this book, we will further discuss the findings of Non-nutritive sweeteners on insulin and weight loss. But for now, let's define Rule #7.

Rule #7: I will eat all of my calories in a 4-5-hour window. This will allow me to have maximal fat burning time throughout the rest of the day. It will allow me to reset my insulin resistance, increase leptin sensitivity, and escape the clutches of metabolic syndrome.

Important Point: I would like you to use 2 weeks to get used to the time-restricted portion of this eating plan. For 2 weeks, let your body acclimate to a 4-5 hours eating window without changing what you eat. Just eat your usual foods. After you feel like your new eating window is natural and easy, you may begin to change components of your diet as outlined in the next chapter. But to begin, it is important to allow your body time to understand that it will no longer be fed around the clock. Don't worry, even during these 2 weeks you will lose weight!

CHAPTER 11: **WHAT TO EAT, WHAT NOT TO EAT**

The Other Half of the Equation

If you simply reduce the time period in which you eat, you will see remarkable changes in your insulin resistance and, subsequently, your weight. This single change, without modification of diets, has led many of my participants to drop 15-20 pounds in one month. Though they ate the same horrible American foods, the effects of a fasting period are amazingly potent.

However, many who use time-restricted eating want to take it further. If you are like me, you want to utilize every possible mechanism to reduce insulin resistance. You want the weight gone, and quickly! To heal my insulin resistance more rapidly, and likewise to lose weight faster, I sought to manipulate my hormones during the period in which I ate. The effects of this manipulation are dramatic, consistent, weight loss, with no risk of "stalling out." Do as I did, and your body will once again sense insulin and leptin *fully*, and your weight will *melt* away. Likewise, your hunger will decrease during both your fasting and eating windows.

The first half of the equation is *when* to eat, but the second half of the equation is equally important. Can we fool our body into thinking we are still fasting, despite wolfing-down the calories? Yes, we can! The second half of the equation is *what to eat* during the feeding hours. If done correctly, you can direct your body to maintain elevated glucagon and fat metabolism while simultaneously eating a steak!

To achieve this effect, we must avoid, at all costs, raising our body's natural insulin levels. Keeping our insulin levels low will allow our bodies to act like they are fasting, despite being in the eating-window. This will exponentially increase how fast our bodies heal, and likewise, how quickly we lose weight.

During our eating window, our insulin levels will rise to meet the demands of the foods we eat. The food becomes a sort of button: Press this button for high insulin, Press this button for no change in insulin. By understanding which foods press which buttons in our body, we can avoid *ever* directing our body to store fat. Using this mechanism, I increased the window during which my body creates ketones from 10 hours, which normally occurs under the 20:4 fasting to eating window, up to 22 hours. This means that in a 24-hour period, there are only 2 hours in which my body is not actively burning fat.

But which foods trigger insulin release? Which contribute to insulin resistance? How are we just finding out about this now? In fact, our knowledge of this is ancient!

Low Carb: The Not So Secret Secret

In 1865, a previously obese man named William Banting wrote a short essay on weight loss. He had the essay printed in a pamphlet, which he then sold for a penny. Banting *was certain* he had found the solution for obesity and was so overcome with his new finding that he tried, as hard as he could, to tell the entire world. The pamphlet was titled, "Letter on Corpulence: Addressed to the Public."

In the pamphlet, Banting describes being one of the very few obese men in his time period. At a meager 5 '5", Banting weighed 202 pounds. This represents a body mass index of 33.6. Today, he would hardly have been noticed in the crowd. But in those days, he stuck out like a sore thumb. He described his experience as an obese man in the 1700s this way,

"I am confident no man laboring under obesity can be quite insensible to the sneers and remarks of the cruel and injudicious public assemblies, public vehicles, or the ordinary street traffic.....therefore he naturally keeps away as much as possible from places where he is likely to be made the object of the taunts and remarks of others."

William Banting, in an effort to reduce his girth, went to multiple physicians. The first, he recalls, advised him to exercise more. Sound familiar?

"I consulted an eminent surgeon, now long deceased, a kind personal friend, who recommended increased bodily exertion before my ordinary daily labours began....It is true I gained muscular vigour, but with it a prodigious appetite, which I was compelled to indulge, and consequently increased in weight, until my kind old friend advised me to forsake the exercise"

Banting experienced what many of us experience today. He took up rowing, exercised each morning, got hungrier, and ultimately gained weight. The second doctor whom Banting consulted recommended calorie restriction. But this too failed. Over the next few years, he sought out and tried many more diets and cures for obesity, but none were effective.

"I consulted other high orthodox authorities (never any inferior adviser), but all in vain. I have tried sea air and bathing in various localities, with much walking exercise ; taken gallons of physic and liquor potassae, advisedly and abundantly ; riding on horseback ; the waters and climate of Leamington many times,... and have spared no trouble nor expense in consultations with the best authorities in the land, giving each and all a fair time for experiment, without any permanent remedy, as the evil still gradually increased."

But finally, Banting found an answer. After these failures, Banting went to a final physician. This physician, among all the others, completely and utterly changed Banting's life. Banting writes,

"...happily, I found the right man, who unhesitatingly sad he believed my ailments were caused principally by corpulence, and prescribed a certain diet...with immense effect and advantage both to my hearing and the decrease of my corpulency"

This physician, ahead of his time, recommended Banting try a low carbohydrate diet.

"The items from which I was advised to abstain as much as possible were : Bread,...milk, sugar, beer, and potatoes, which had been the main (and, I thought, innocent) elements of my existence, ... These, said my excellent adviser, contain starch and saccharine matter, tending to create fat, and should be avoided altogether...."

The results were tremendous. Banting recounts,

"I have not felt so well as now for the last twenty years. Have suffered no inconvenience whatever in the probational remedy. Am reduced many inches in bulk, and 35 lbs. in weight in thirty-eight weeks....take ordinary exercise freely, without the slightest inconvenience. My sight is restored – my hearing improved. My other bodily ailments are ameliorated ; indeed, almost past into matter of history."

William Banting found, through experimentation with different doctors and their recommendations, that only a low carbohydrate diet decreased his hunger, increased his energy, and finally dropped his weight. However, neither Banting nor his doctor understood the mechanism of why this dietary changed caused weight loss. There was no understanding of insulin: glucagon ratio, nor of insulin resistance. Yet he had found a way, through diet, to heal his own.

After William Banting, low carbohydrate diets for obesity were common-place throughout the late 1800s and early 1900s. Low carbohydrate diets were taught commonly in the medical schools of the early 1900s as the definitive cure for excess fat.

In the 1950s, women's magazines boasted the knowledge that carbohydrates are fattening. Mothers taught their daughters to avoid sweets and breads to lose weight. Even recognized medical journals touted the knowledge.

As early as 1923 it was known that the pancreas (where insulin is secreted) was necessary for obesity. "A functionally intact pancreas is necessary for fattening...", stated Wilhelm Falta, physician and author of *Endocrine Diseases*, a 1923 work on obesity in the era. But what was it about the pancreas, and carbohydrates which caused this obesity? It remained poorly understood. Low carbohydrate diets, however, continued to reign.

In 1951 Raymond Greene, in his book, *The Practice of Endocrinology*, recommended the abstinence from bread, flour products, cereals, potatoes and sweets for the curing of obesity. He advocated his patients eat as much as they want of meat, green vegetables, eggs, cheese, and fruit, with the exception of bananas and grapes (which have considerable carbohydrate content).

In 1957 Hilde Bruch, a leading childhood obesity researcher, wrote, "The great progress in dietary control of obesity was the recognition that meat...was not fat producing...but that it was the innocent foodstuffs, such as bread and sweets, which lead to obesity."

In 1958 Dr. Richard Mackarness published *Eat Fat and Grow Slim*, in which he stated carbohydrates, and not calories, were the true culprit in weight gain.

In 1961, Herman Taller published a book called *Calories Don't Count* explaining why high-fat, high-calorie diets worked to lose weight. He was the first to recognize that carbohydrates stimulate insulin, leading to fat storage.

In 1963 famous endocrinologist George Cahill further tied weight gain to insulin. He famously wrote, "Carbohydrate is driving insulin is driving fat."

In 1965 Rosalyn Yalow, a Nobel prize-winning American medical physicist recognized that the release of fatty acids from fat cells, and subsequent weight loss, "requires only the negative stimulus of insulin deficiency." In other words, less insulin, less fat.

Even Dr. Spock, celebrated child-rearing expert wrote, "Rich desserts and the amount of plain starchy foods (cereals, breads, potatoes) taken is what determines, in the case of most people, how much they gain or lose."

If the whole world knew that refined carbohydrates and sweets (flours, starches, sugars and today corn syrup) cause obesity, what changed?

The Almighty Calorie

In the early 1900s, an obsession with a newly discovered technology, the calorimeter, emerged. With the invention of the calorimeter in 1860, scientists were, for the first time, able to measure the number of "calories" in a gram of fat, protein, or carbohydrate. The science became cutting edge and high tech. Following this invention, theories surfaced that explained obesity as simply a problem of too many calories eaten, while too few calories were expended. This sounded scientific and intelligent. Over the next 100 years, people began to blame calories as a whole, instead of trying to explain how each macronutrient may affect the body differently.

This model, which theorizes "all calories are equal," has led us to where we are today. Believing that 200 calories of gummy bears are the same as 200 calories of T-bone steak has created a generation of suffering, obese, and hopeless human beings. However, until the 1970s, despite emerging calorie science, Americans still knew better: it was the carbs which caused obesity. So surely something else changed? Indeed, it did!

As we discussed previously, in 1956, Ancel Keys jumped on the scene. He had arrived to save us from our normal weights and shepherd us into the land of obscene obesity. He demonized saturated fats, convinced an entire world they cause heart disease, and moved our society from anti-carbohydrate to anti-fat. The knowledge that refined carbohydrates cause obesity was forgotten, despite 200 hundred years of effective dieting. Overnight, fat was the single macronutrient to blame for all of the world's problems. What a shame!

Low Carb High Fat, But What About Protein?

Today, the "Keto" diet is very popular. The term "Keto" stands for Ketogenic and endorses a ratio of macronutrients, high in dietary fat, which favors the creation of ketones. The idea is that metabolism of ketones as the body's primary fuel, rather than glucose, then induces the body to utilize stored fat, as well as dietary fat, for energy. Sounds good so far! In the medical world, the popularized term "Keto" has been replaced with the designation "Low Carb High Fat" or LCHF.

But what is a truly ketogenic diet? Indeed, a quick web search will bring up hundreds of variations on "Keto" diets. Ketogenic food recipes are everywhere, but it is hard to discern what foods are truly helpful versus harmful for our worsening insulin resistance. Who even came up with the idea anyway?

In truth, the term "ketogenic diet" dates back 100 years. In 1921, Dr. Russel Wilder coined the term ketogenic diet for a diet which reduces carbohydrates and increases fat as a means of raising ketones in the blood. The diet was originally invented as a way to treat epileptic children.

The Ketogenic or LCHF diet is effective. It can lead to both lowered insulin resistance, as well as lowered weight. But among popular ketogenic diet circles, some stringent recommendations are proliferated. Are its stringent recommendations necessary? The diet prescribes a macronutrient ratio in which 75% of calories are consumed as fat. Generally, 20% of calories are consumed as protein, and 5% are consumed as carbohydrate. The standing recommendation is to maintain this macronutrient balance or risk creating too much glucose and falling out of ketosis. For me, this is simply too complex.

Surely God did not design our bodies to come with a calculator, working out our fat to protein macronutrient ratio? If God meant us to do this, why are there no overweight animals in nature except the ones who eat human food? Where are the macronutrient graphs for the bunny rabbits? Or the wolves? Or the majestic Zebra?

Because of a fear of glucose and the possibility of knocking one's self "out of ketosis," the modern ketogenic diet is ***terrified*** of protein. The standing reasoning is that the body, through gluconeogenesis, can convert too much protein into glucose, thus stalling ketosis. The glucose created through the digestion of protein, they theorize, has as much potential for weight gain as a diet rich in carbohydrates. Likewise, they cite studies that show protein consumption can lead to insulin release, thus inhibiting ketogenesis and leading to weight gain. For this reason, they recommend 75-80% fat as the primary dietary macronutrient. This leads to bizarre behavior. One ketogenic enthusiast I know often drinks tablespoons of olive oil poured straight from the bottle. Yikes!

Protein definitely raises insulin. It also has the potential to be converted to glucose. But are the fears that it will stall weight loss justified?

Interestingly, modern ketogenic enthusiasts often remember the insulin portion of the hormone equation, but they forget about the glucagon. The question the modern ketogenic enthusiasts **should ask** is not "can protein convert to glucose and cause insulin release," but rather, "what effect does protein have on the insulin: glucagon ratio?"

Dog Gone It!

As we discussed in our chapter on Insulin and Glucagon, in 1971, a phenomenal study was performed with canine subjects. This study, perhaps more important than any other study of macronutrients ever done, studied the insulin: glucagon ratio of canine subjects after intravenous boluses of protein. What they found has huge implications for Low Carb High Fat (ketogenic) diets.

After fasting, the dogs were given intravenous amino acids, the smallest component of protein. After the bolus of amino acids, the dogs' insulin levels increased, just as modern ketogenic science predicts. Insulin increased from 1.0 to 2.0 relative units, doubling the levels of the fasted state. This is what the ketogenic diet enthusiasts fear: an increase in insulin. But what they miss is what happened to Glucagon. Stunning the scientists, the Glucagon level elevated 4 times as much as insulin. As insulin increased from 1.0 to 2.0 relative units, glucagon elevated from 1.0 to 4.0! This created a net decrease in the insulin: glucagon ratio, with a subsequent ratio of 0.5. This is lower than the fasted state!

The scientists concluded that the pancreas of these canine subjects recognized a need for insulin to transport amino acids across the cell membrane. However, there is a dilemma for the body. Insulin causes a decrease in circulating blood glucose. If the pancreases of these canine subjects simply dumped insulin, without any source of carbohydrates, the effect would be a dangerously low blood glucose, seizure, and death.

So, the body has to do two contradictory things at once. On the one hand, it must secrete insulin to utilize the amino acids. On the other hand, it must protect against hypoglycemia (low blood sugar). The answer to this conundrum is to elevate *both* insulin and glucagon, with glucagon in the predominant hormonal position. An increase in both hormones, with glucagon predominant, leads to the transport of amino acids across the cell membrane via insulin, as well as the conversion of amino acids to small amounts of glucose, with the simultaneous maintenance of blood glucose levels at normal levels.

But for our study, this leads to another fantastic result. At a ratio superior to fasting, protein in the absence of carbohydrates leads to a glucagon spike. In the presence of high glucagon, the body begins to burn fat stores and generate ketones. And so, ketogenesis elevates after protein consumption! Modern ketogenic diets, with their instructions to keep protein macronutrient ratios at 20%, completely miss the point!

Because of this amazing benefit of protein, and contrary to modern ketogenic (LCHF) advice, I want you to think of protein as your *primary* macronutrient. Do not fear it at all. Do not trouble yourself with 20%, or 80%, or any percent. Simply follow the rules outlined below, and throw away the calculator.

Carnivorous Carnitine, Destroyer of Fat

Protein has another amazing benefit. Protein is rich in a substance called L-Carnitine. This amino acid has a very special job! In the body, L-Carnitine binds to fatty acids in the cells and holds their hand as they cross the membrane of the mitochondria. L-Carnitine is essential for fatty acids to be burned away.

In the mitochondria, the body burns stored body fat for energy and heat, deleting that fatty acid from your body forever. Without L-Carnitine, a traffic jam develops. Fat is unable to efficiently enter the mitochondria and stacks up in the cytoplasmic jelly of the cell.

In 2013, researchers evaluated the L-Carnitine levels present in both normal-weight and obese women. The women with BMI < 18.5 (very thin) had significantly *higher* serum L-Carnitine levels, whereas the women with BMI > 29.9 (obese) had significantly *lower* serum L-Carnitine levels. This means that the average thin person has a higher amount of L-Carnitine, necessary for fat transport, than their obese counterpart!

In a 2016 review of the literature on Carnitine, it was found that people deficient in L-Carnitine had significantly reduced capacity to lose weight. Likewise, the researchers, reviewing 9 trials and 911 participants, determined that subjects who received Carnitine supplementation consistently lost more weight than those who did not. As you can see, to become efficient fat burners, we must have high levels of L-Carnitine.

So where do we get Carnitine? All animal meats and eggs contain Carnitine. But without exception, the highest source of this amazing molecule is in red meat. Beef contains carnitine levels 1000% higher than chicken or fish. A 4-ounce beef steak has an estimated 162 mg of carnitine. A 4-ounce chicken breast, by comparison, contains 5 mg. Bread contains less than 1 mg. For this reason, as well as the glucagonergic effect noted in canines, a person should ideally begin their eating window each day with a meal rich in protein. And more ideally, a meal rich in red meat. This was so important to my weight loss success that we must pause to define our eighth rule:

Rule# 8: Each day, I will begin my eating window with a large protein bolus. When possible, I will eat red meat to increase my carnitine levels.

Carbohydrates are NOT Evil, But We Have to Heal!

The Ketogenic diet is likewise obvious in its loathing of carbohydrates, and for good reason: they knock you out of ketosis. But do they always? Are all carbohydrates the same? My own findings have not shown this. The things which have raised my blood sugar most dramatically, and caused my fat-burning to stop are the carbohydrates invented by humankind. Carbohydrates invented by God generally affect me very minimally.

Anyone who tells you we must be low carbohydrate to maintain thinness is fooling themselves. In 1960, almost everyone was thin. Yet there was a toaster in almost every American home. Do not think for a moment that I believe the 1960s American was low carb! However, as you have seen throughout this book, our insulin sensitivity has been destroyed by many different foods since 1960. Vegetable oils, Fructose, the removal of fiber, and the general bastardization of our normal food supply has poisoned our systems. We are now insulin resistant, unlike our 1960s counterpart. And for this reason, we must become low-carbohydrate. To heal our system, we must give up things which our 1960s ancestors enjoyed, in order to return to a state of insulin sensitivity similar to theirs.

The breads, the cereals, the processed and refined carbohydrates of our generation, as well as the added oils and fructose, are the guilty parties, not the macronutrient "carbohydrate" at large. Some modern low carb and ketogenic diets throw the proverbial baby out with the bathwater. Not all carbohydrates are bad. Not all carbohydrates prevent ketosis and the metabolism of fat. Not all carbohydrates cause insulin resistance! And, as a type 1 diabetic, not all raise my blood glucose significantly, nor require much insulin at all.

With that said, as obese Americans, we are no longer in a place to eat a diet rich in carbohydrates. We must first heal our insulin resistance. In the same way that I, as a type 1 diabetic, can never partake of foods rich in refined carbohydrates, an obese American, insulin resistant and pre-diabetic, must view themselves as having been diagnosed with a disease. This disease requires dietary guidelines and treatment. The treatment is a low carbohydrate diet designed to lower insulin levels and reduce body fat.

Carbohydrates are not evil, but insulin resistance is! For this reason, we require a two-phase diet. In the first phase, we will heal our bodies of the terrible havoc unleashed on them by the American diet. We must reverse decades of insulin resistance which began in your body after your first bite of American food.

In the first phase, we will use our eating window to eat only foods which raise blood glucose negligibly. The idea will be to mimic a type 1 diabetic, very conscious of the effect each food has on blood glucose. If a food raises blood sugar enough to necessitate taking exogenous insulin (insulin shot), then it will, by its nature, require a non-diabetic's pancreas to secrete insulin in the same way. In this way, I am your guinea pig. You cannot see what each food does to your insulin secretion, but I can. I am your human litmus test.

After returning to a healthy weight, and normal blood glucose (HbA1C), you may (if you wish) begin phase two of the eating plan. This phase will re-introduce the healthy carbohydrates which God made for you. These foods, including fruits and starchier vegetables, will raise your blood glucose more than the foods in phase 1. However, they will not produce the long-lasting insulin resistance and the spiral of obesity which the American diet has caused within us all.

Let's look at the foods to eat, and avoid, in each phase. By eating only foods which do not raise blood glucose, your body will stay in a state of ketone generation and weight loss during almost all of the 24 hours in a day. Get ready to lose weight!

Phase 1: What to Eat

During your eating window, you may **eat as much as you like** of the following foods:

1. **Low Carbohydrate Vegetables**: Almost all vegetables are allowed, except for those with significant starch content. Vegetables which will not increase blood glucose or insulin include:

    a. Arugula, Artichoke, Broccoli, Brussel Sprouts, Cabbage, Carrots, Cauliflower, Collard Greens, Cucumber, Eggplant, Green Beans, Lettuce (any type), Mushrooms, Onions, Olives, Spinach, Squash, Zucchini, and All "Cruciferous" Vegetables

Each of these vegetables was tested against my own blood glucose and raised it almost insignificantly. If a food did not make the list, it ratcheted my blood glucose into unhealthy ranges or required significant insulin to maintain blood glucose.

2. **Fruits**: Only the fruits which minimally raise blood glucose are allowed. These include:

    a. Avocado, Blackberries, Blueberries, Raspberries, Strawberries, Tomatoes
    b. Lemon and Lime are fine for cooking (as well as lemon/lime juice in small amounts for cooking)

3. **Fats**:

    a. Butter, Olive Oil, Avocado Oil, Coconut Oil, Lard, Beef Tallow

Fats and oils have almost no effect on blood glucose. This is generally true of all oils; however, what is important here is to eradicate "vegetable oils" from the diet. These are found in almost every modern American food. Have no fear of saturated fats, as these are your body's preferred fats.

4. **Protein**:

    a.   All Animal Meats and Eggs

The only requirement is to avoid any meats which have been processed with sugar, such as canned meats or cured meats. These meats will generally include the trifecta of vegetable oils, sugar and/or corn syrup. For example, it is very difficult to find a salami or bacon that has not been cured with sugar. If you are able to find a cured meat without some form of sugar, then it is allowed.

If you have the means, I highly suggest grass-fed beef, rather than corn-fed. Grass-fed animals have lower levels of Omega-6 fatty acids and higher levels of Omega-3 fatty acids. This is a recommendation, not a rule. (Grass Fed Beef is twice the price)

5. **Dairy**:

    a.   Cheese, Heavy Whipping Cream, Butter, Sour Cream, Cream Cheese

As far as the rest of the above list, make sure, once again, that no sugar has been added, and that no vegetable oils have been added to your product.

Phase 1: What Not to Eat

During your eating window, *avoid the foods listed below*. Each will elevate your insulin levels, leading to body fat.

1. **Refined Carbohydrates**:

    a.   Added Sugar: Any products with sugar added (listed in the ingredients as one of the 56 names of sugar - see chapter 4 -) are to be avoided.

b. Refined Carbohydrates: Breads, Pasta, Cereals, and Grains (Corn, Rice, Wheat, Millet, Quinoa, Cuscus, Oats, Barley).

c. Avoid any products with flour.

All of these foods are refined in modern America to a degree unseen throughout history. They raise my blood glucose quickly and to a devastating degree. I often require multiple large boluses of insulin to conquer the blood glucose effect of these foods.

2. **Fruits**:

a. All fruits beside Blueberries, Blackberries, Raspberries, Strawberries, Tomato, and Avocado (as well as lemon and lime juice for cooking) are to be avoided in Phase 1

Fruits are healthy and wonderful. But not in Phase 1 of this insulin resistance diet. We are trying to heal you of the disease of insulin resistance! Until you have healed, fruits are limited to those above.

3. **Vegetables**:

a. All starchy vegetables should be avoided. These include corn, potatoes, parsnips, sweet potato. A simple way to recognize a starchy vegetable is where it grows. "Root Vegetables" are often high in carbohydrate.

b. Avoid "tomato sauces" or "spaghetti sauces" during Phase 1. These sauces start off as healthy tomatoes but boil down to almost pure glucose. They raise my blood sugar quickly and keep it elevated for about 24 hours, requiring large doses of insulin. (A bit of sugar-free ketchup is fine in Phase 1)

4. **Nuts**:
   a.   All nuts should be avoided in phase 1.

Contrary to popular opinion about nuts on a Ketogenic diet, I have found that nuts raise my blood glucose extraordinarily fast. There are considerable amounts of carbohydrates in nuts, and very few people can eat only a handful of them. Moreover, the high Omega-6 fatty acid content of nuts will delay the healing of your insulin resistance. Avoid nuts until phase 2.

   b.   **Nut Flours**: Almond flour, Coconut Flour, and other nut flours are to be avoided.

Despite seeming low carbohydrate, nut flours raise blood glucose very quickly. They are heavily refined, high in Omega-6 fatty acids, and eaten in extremely high quantities (almond flour pizza dough, for example). Avoid nut flours altogether.

5. **Legumes**:
   a.   Avoid all legumes except green beans.

Legumes are often referred to as "beans." Beans raise my blood glucose and insulin demand quickly. Legumes include peanuts, peas, soybeans, lentils, chickpeas, pinto beans, navy beans, lima beans, kidney beans, black-eyed peas. Green beans, however, do not raise my blood glucose and are fine!

6. **Fats**:

   a.   No Processed Seed (or Vegetable) Oils: These include Soybean oil, Canola oil, Corn oil, Safflower oil, Sunflower oil, Grapeseed oil, Peanut Oil, Sesame Oil, Linseed Oil, Cottonseed Oil.

The list grows longer every day. All of these are heavily processed unnatural oils. The effects of these oils have been discussed throughout this book and include increased insulin resistance, increased obesity, elevated cancer risk, gallbladder pathology, increased inflammation, and a host of other harmful effects. Only use high Oleic Fatty Acids when oil is required, such as olive or avocado oil.

    b. No Margarine or Shortening: Just use butter or animal fat!

Do not accept any butter imitation or animal fat imitation. When solid fats are required, just use real butter! In the next chapter, we will discuss the amazing benefits of saturated fat. Do not believe the lies about saturated fat; these animal fats are a *key* to health. The unhealthy fats are the ones made in a factory.

    c. Beware of "butter sprays," as these are often 100% soybean oil.

7. **Protein**:

    a. Avoid cured meats and deli meats: These are often filled with sugar, corn syrup, and/or nitrates.

8. **Dairy**:

    a. Avoid Milk: Milk has a very high glycemic load and will raise your blood glucose and insulin very quickly and powerfully.

Milk is often used by paramedics as a drink to reverse severe low blood sugar (hypoglycemia) in diabetics. Milk, as I have experienced firsthand, raises my blood glucose faster than a can of cola or a glass of orange juice. The sugar is healthy, in the form of lactose, but nonetheless it converts to glucose in your bloodstream very quickly and should be avoided while we are trying to heal our insulin resistance.

    b. Avoid Yogurt (Greek, Plain, or Flavored)

    c.   Avoid Ricotta and Cottage Cheese (both are high in sugar)

    d.   Avoid any dairy products with added sugar, even if approved above.

    e.   Avoid added sugars or "starches" which may be hidden in pre-shredded cheese. Shredded cheese is often coated in starch to reduce caking. In the Cimino home, we buy cheese in blocks and shred it ourselves.

What the Heck Can I Eat?

I know what you are thinking: "What the heck can I eat on this diet?" Often, looking at a list of do's and don'ts seems onerous and restrictive. It seems extreme. But it isn't! After getting used to phase one, you will see the elimination of refined carbohydrates, sugar, and vegetable oil from your diet changes you. You will begin to feel internally cleaner; your system will run amazingly well. And moreover, you will lose weight! For years, you have been pouring sugar and chemicals down your gas tank, raising your insulin to ridiculous levels. Your weight has ballooned, and perhaps now they are calling you "pre-diabetic." The simple changes above can reverse and heal all of that. And let me tell you, it can be delicious as well!

Do not perseverate on the list of do's and don'ts, but rather think about what is *allowed* with this style of eating. Picture one of my favorite lunches: a freshly grilled hamburger covered in cheddar cheese and avocado, with a romaine side salad chocked full of diced egg and shredded cheddar cheese, all smothered in homemade ranch dressing. On the side are low carbohydrate fried pickles, dipped in ranch. My mouth is watering now! And what effect does it have on my blood glucose? Almost none!

Eating the foods above, I have lowered my monthly insulin requirement from 7000 units to around 650 units per month. I likewise lost 116 lbs. Though you will not be able to calculate how much less insulin your own body needs (unless you are diabetic), you will see dramatic effects in weight and general health which will indicate that the *exact* same thing is happening in your own body. You will reverse *decades* of insulin resistance, leptin resistance, and obesity.

In phase two, life gets even better.

Phase 2:

Phase 2, as we have stated above, is marked by one of two scenarios. If you are not a diabetic, then this phase will begin when you have fully reached your goal weight. The reaching of your goal weight will indicate you are healed of insulin resistance and may begin to introduce carbohydrate-rich foods into your diet. Similarly, if you have type 2 diabetes, the eradication of all diabetes medications (by your physician), as well as the return to normal weight, will indicate that Phase 2 is ready to begin.

In Phase 2, we will allow back some foods which do raise blood sugar, but not enough to restart the cycle of insulin resistance, diabetes, and obesity. Should you find you begin to gain back any weight, simply revert to phase 1. For each macronutrient, I will include the foods allowed in phase 1, plus some additions.

Phase 2

1. **Fruits and Vegetables**: In phase 2, all vegetables and fruits are now allowed.

    a. Low Carbohydrate Vegetables: Avocado, Arugula, Broccoli, Brussel Sprouts, Cabbage, Cauliflower, Carrots, Collard Greens, Cucumber, Eggplant, Green Beans, Lettuce (Romaine or Iceberg), Olives, Spinach,

Tomato, Zucchini continue to be allowed and encouraged in phase 2

    b. Starchy Vegetables: White Potato, Sweet Potato, Whole Kernel Corn are allowed in phase 2.

    c. Fruits: All fruits are allowed in Phase 2

2. **Refined Grains**: Continue to avoid refined cereals and grains in Phase 2. The level of processing in commercial grains (regardless of whole wheat or white) is high enough to begin pushing your insulin resistance upward again.

3. **Fats**: Fats are unchanged in Phase 2

    a. Butter, Olive Oil, Avocado Oil, Coconut Oil, Lard, Beef Tallow

    b. Continue to avoid Seed Oils in phase 2!

4. **Protein**: Protein sources are unchanged in phase 2

    a. All Animal Meats and Eggs

    b. Continue to avoid nitrates and added sugar

5. **Dairy**:

a. Cheese, Heavy Whipping Cream, Butter, Sour Cream, Greek Yogurt, Cream Cheese

b. Milk is **_allowed_** in phase 2. The sugar in milk is lactose, which your body can handle easily. With normal insulin sensitivity, this will not harm you.

c. Ricotta and Cottage Cheese are **_allowed_** in Phase 2.

d. Continue to avoid any dairy products with added sugar.

6. **Nuts**:

   a. All nuts are **_allowed_** in Phase 2.

   b. However, continue to avoid "Nut Flours"

7. **Legumes**:

   a. All Legumes such as peanuts, peas, and beans are **_allowed_** in Phase 2

Phase 2 is certainly less restrictive. The idea here is that you are still keeping your insulin sensitivity at bay by eating only foods God has made for you, which contain both natural fiber and many other micronutrients which promote excellent health. Phase one is more restrictive only because we are trying to undo so much damage which the American diet has wrought on you.

In Phase 2, you should continue your decided time-window for eating, though you may expand your time window slightly. If you prefer, you may adjust your eating window from 4 hours to 6 or even 8 hours. You must, however, continue to restrict feeding to a dedicated portion of the day. The benefits of time-restricted eating and your hours of fasting should persist for your whole life! You were built for them!

As indicated above, nut flours should be avoided. In modern low-carbohydrate, high-fat culture, it has become popular to replace wheat flour with almond flour or coconut flour in an effort to make many of the foods (such as pizza) which people miss on a low-carbohydrate diet. Unfortunately, these flours are highly refined and can raise blood glucose levels very quickly. These nut flours have very high levels of Omega-6 fatty acids which have been shown to induce inflammation and subsequently insulin and leptin resistance. I avoid them. You should too.

Let us look now at a 3-day sample of my diet. My own eating window begins at 4 pm and ends at 8 pm. During that time, I eat luxurious, beautiful meals. I do not calorie count. I eat as much as I want until I am completely full. Neither do I exercise, and yet I have lost 116 pounds and lowered my insulin requirement dramatically. My A1C is in the non-diabetic range (despite having type 1 diabetes!), and my energy levels and emotional state have never been better.

Day 1:

Fasting Period:

Black Coffee with Splenda, Diet Soda

4 PM Lunch:

Cheese Burger on Egg Bread, Zucchini Fries with Sugar-Free Ketchup

7 PM Dinner:

Garlic Pot Roast, Cauli-Mash, Sautéed Spinach

7:30 PM Dessert:

"Naked" Cheesecake

Day 2:

Fasting Period:

Black Coffee with Splenda, Diet Soda

4 PM Lunch:

4-egg Cheese Omelet, 6 Slices of Bacon, 2 Slices of "Toastless" French Toast

7 PM Dinner:

Margarita Cauliflower Pizza, Greek Salad with Olives and Feta

7:30 PM Dessert:

Coconut Oil Chocolate, Coffee creamed with Heavy Whipping Cream

Day 3:

Fasting Period:

Black Coffee with Splenda, Diet Soda

4 PM Lunch:

Tuna Salad dressed with Mayo on Romaine Lettuce, Dill Pickle, Sliced Tomato with Mozzarella and Olive Oil Vinaigrette

7 PM Dinner:

Ground Beef Taco Bowl with Avocado Guaca-Salsa topping

7:30 PM Dessert:

Raspberry Low Carb Ice Cream

Other common eating-window snacks: String cheese, Hard Boiled or Deviled Eggs, Raw Veggies and Ranch

Rule #9: I will eat a low-carbohydrate diet. Of this diet, I will eat as much as I want, without calorie counting. Likewise, I will not count macronutrient ratios. I will prefer protein over all other macronutrients.

Important Point: For the first two weeks of these food changes, you may feel much the same as Dr. Schwatka when he switched to eating primarily reindeer meat in the arctic. While your body switches from a lifetime of glucose metabolism and ramps up ketone metabolism, you may feel run down. Please do not give up! After two weeks of eating "low carb," your body will become efficient at burning fat for fuel. You will feel energized! Your belly fat will shrink, and your energy levels and endurance will increase! Even your cravings will change. You will begin to desire protein and fats, with little interest in carbohydrates.

Another Important Point: When eating a low carbohydrate diet, make sure to eat plenty of salt. Insulin increases salt reabsorption in the kidneys. With lower insulin levels, your body will waste salt. So, unless you have been advised to maintain a low-sodium diet, don't be shy when seasoning your food.

CHAPTER 12: **CHOLESTEROL**

A Persevering Fear

One of the most common concerns that I hear regarding a diet high in saturated fat and animal meat is on the issue of cholesterol. Won't saturated fat elevate my cholesterol and increase my risk for heart disease? Nothing could be farther from the truth! Once again, America has been fed half-truths, which do not tell the whole story.

The tremendous fear of saturated fat which pervades all levels of American culture are unfounded. My own cholesterol levels, after eating in the manner described to you in the last two chapters, dropped in *half*. My personal physician was stunned. After eating animal fat and butter, with daily red meat, he no longer needed to place me on a cholesterol medication!

For well over 50 years, saturated fats have been vilified in America. Starting in 1977, following the work of Ancel Keys, the official edict from the nutritionists and physicians on high was "reduce your saturated fat intake from 40% to 30%, and favor poly-unsaturated fats". We were told to replace our diets with seed oils and to reduce all animal and saturated fats to stave off heart disease. But has it actually worked? The data may surprise you.

A Slowly Sinking Ship

As a physician, I hear constantly from both patients and other physicians, "I won't eat bacon, too much saturated fat." And, "My doctor tells me my cholesterol is too high, she just started me on a statin. I'm not allowed to eat butter." Or perhaps even more unbelievably, "I only eat the egg whites. I'm on a low cholesterol diet." And yet these same individuals eat their egg whites with a side of refined white toast and jam!

As you can see, even six decades later, Ancel Keys dominates the minds of both physicians and the lay public. That's a powerful influence indeed. But if all of the fear of saturated fats started with Ancel Keys, has the science since 1956 proven he was right? Or does it show a different picture?

Ancel Key's seminal work, the "Seven Countries Study," purported to show a clear correlation between diets rich in saturated fat and heart disease. But did it actually prove anything at all? LDL cholesterol, recently discovered in the time of Ancel Keys, was found to be higher in individuals who ate higher amounts of saturated fat. LDL cholesterol, it was believed at the time, led to heart disease. So, without scientific understanding or significant evidence, the connection was made that saturated fat *must* cause heart disease.

Scientists of the last four generations have not been lazy in trying to prove this theory. No, in fact, they have done everything they could to prove Ancel Keys was correct. Scientists just want saturated fat to be bad for you *so badly*! Unfortunately, after over 100 billion dollars in large, well-funded studies, *none* can prove that saturated fats lead to a higher incidence of heart disease. Some studies even show the opposite!

In science, we have something called a "meta-analysis." A meta-analysis compiles the results of multiple studies into one large scientific review, in an attempt to boil down the noise of multiple, sometimes conflicting, papers. Meta-analyses represent the most comprehensive way to review large amounts of data, collected throughout decades of research studies. Over the last 20 years, many large meta-analyses have been conducted reviewing all and any evidence of saturated fat's roll in heart disease. Let me show you a few of their findings:

1.   "…no significant evidence for concluding that dietary

saturated fat is associated with an increased risk of Coronary Heart Disease or Cardiovascular Disease"

2. "There were no clear effects of dietary fat changes on total mortality or cardiovascular mortality…"

3. "Saturated fats are not associated with all-cause mortality, Cardiovascular Disease, Coronary Heart Disease, Ischemic Stroke, or type 2 diabetes."

4. "…no mortality benefit for the intervention group in the full randomized cohort or for any prespecified subgroup. There was a 22% higher risk of death for each 0.78 mmol/L reduction in serum-cholesterol."

5. "…replacing Saturated Fatty Acid with mostly [vegetable oil] is unlikely to reduce Coronary Heart Disease events, Coronary Heart Disease mortality, or total mortality. The suggestion of benefits reported in earlier meta-analyses is due to the inclusion of inadequately controlled trials."

None of these meta-analyses found any link between saturated animal fats and increased risk of death, heart disease, stroke, or any other negative consequence. In the fourth review listed above, there was even an increased risk of death from the reduction of cholesterol! The take away from these reviews, as well as countless others, is that saturated fat is *fine for you*! All of our efforts to replace saturated fats with factory-made vegetable oils were in vain. These supposed experts stole bacon and butter from us, *for no darn reason!*

What is "Cholesterol" Anyway?

But what about cholesterol? Isn't cholesterol bad? What is it, anyway? Today we throw around the world cholesterol, but almost no one understands what it actually is. Cholesterol itself is a molecule which makes up 30% of your cell walls. It is vital to life. It forms the precursor to your sex hormones, your stress hormones, Vitamin D, as well as a myriad of other vital chemicals in your body.
Most of the cholesterol in your body comes from your body itself.

Indeed, your own body produces around 70% of your cholesterol, with diet contributing the other 30%. However, in medicine, "cholesterol" does not actually mean cholesterol. Confusing, right?

The term "cholesterol" is a trick of nomenclature. When your doctor discusses your "cholesterol" or your "lipid panel," he or she is referring to something called "lipoproteins" and not to the actual molecule of cholesterol. Lipoproteins, including LDL and HDL, are the transport molecules for fatty acids in your bloodstream.

As you know, oil and water do not mix. When God designed your body, He thought of this. His answer was to make large spherical molecules called lipoproteins, composed of phospholipids (which dissolve in water) and protein. These lipoproteins essentially form a bubble, encasing, and packing fatty acids in their core. By transporting the fat in a structure made of protein and phospholipids, the body is able to overcome the problem of oil and water separation. These molecules, then, are a vital part of your body's processes, despite the vilification in modern medicine.

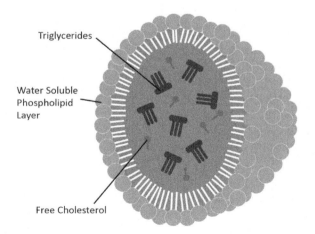

When your doctor tests your cholesterol, he or she tests the markers of Total Cholesterol, HDL, LDL, and Triglycerides. Total cholesterol is a measure of all of the lipoproteins in your bloodstream at the moment your blood is drawn. Triglyceride level is a measure of the fatty acids in your bloodstream. This is usually tested after a period of fasting, as something you recently ate can affect it. None of these molecules, however, is true cholesterol (as you would find in an egg yolk). These molecules, rather, are carrier molecules which live in the bloodstream. Their job is to transport fat and cholesterol around the body.

HDL stands for High Density Lipoprotein. It is "high density" because it has less fat inside it, and is a smaller molecule. It is, therefore, denser with protein, and smaller overall. This is the portion of your cholesterol which is thought to transport fatty acids away from your arteries and back to the liver. This is generally accepted to be the "good cholesterol" because it is moving fats away from your circulation.

LDL stands for low density lipoprotein. This molecule is low density, as its name implies. The reason its density is low is because the molecule is loaded up and "fluffy" with fats. It is generally thought to transport fatty acids from the liver to the circulation. The assumption became that this molecule *must* be bad, as it is moving fat towards your bloodstream, and must deposit (it was assumed) at least some of that fat on the walls of the arteries. It has come to be villainized more than any other particle in the "cholesterol panel." When Ancel Keys tried to correlate cholesterol to heart disease, he blamed LDL.

So, LDL is bad, and HDL is good. So Simple! Doctors have been using this paradigm for decades. They prescribe statins (cholesterol-lowering medications) at the drop of a hat based on this simple understanding. But is it that simple? Modern findings have proven, as usual, it isn't!

LDL: The Double Agent

LDL, as it turns out, comes in two forms. The first form is known as Pattern A LDL and the second as Pattern B LDL. Pattern A LDL includes LDL-1 and LDL-2. Pattern B LDL includes LDL-3, LDL-4, LDL-5, LDL-6, and LDL-7. As you can see, there is much more differentiation than just "LDL."

In modern medicine, almost no physician will test your LDL

for the composition of pattern A or pattern B. The result you obtain from a standard American lipid panel is simply "LDL." What's worse: the LDL on your doctor's blood panel isn't even truly tested! Rather, it is estimated based on the other results of the test.

The difference between these two "Patterns" of LDL is oxidization. Pattern A is "non-oxidized," whereas Pattern B is oxidized. Oxidization is simply the attachment of oxygen molecules to the molecules of the lipoprotein. Think of rust on a car. On a rusty car, the metal has "oxidized."

As it turns out, Pattern A has been shown to be entirely harmless to the human system. Pattern B LDL, on the other hand, is associated with increased heart disease and cardiovascular risk.

A 2016 review of multiple studies involving both patterns of LDL found that a high concentration of Pattern B LDL alongside a low concentration of Pattern A LDL is associated with a significantly greater Coronary Heart Disease risk. Likewise, A 1994 study showed that elevated Pattern B LDL correlated to an increased risk of heart disease of 450%.

A 1992 Study at Stanford showed that Oxidized LDL (Pattern B), and not Pattern A, is implicated in the sequence of events leading to fatty streak formation (arterial clogging) in the arterial intima (inner layer of the heart arteries). They noted that increased oxidative modifications of Pattern B LDL contribute to increased atherosclerosis in humans whose cholesterol profile is rich in Pattern B.

A 2017 study showed that Pattern B LDL has a greater atherogenic potential than that of all other LDL subfractions. The researchers noted that Pattern B LDL readily undergoes multiple modifications which lead to atherosclerosis and arterial clogging, including further oxidation, glycation, and inflammation.

As pattern B is clearly associated with higher heart disease and cardiovascular risk, what determines whether a person has Pattern A or Pattern B LDL? To evaluate this, we must look at the effects of diet on these two types.

It's Our Food, Of Course!

Which foods make Pattern A go up? Which foods make Pattern B go up? Let's look at the research!

A 2005 study showed that increased dietary carbohydrates, particularly simple sugars and starches with high glycemic index, increase levels of Pattern B LDL, primarily by mechanisms that involve increasing plasma triglyceride concentrations.

A 2016 review repeated this finding, showing that many lines of evidence have implicated sugars more than saturated fat in the creation of Pattern B LDL. So strong were their findings that the researchers urged dietary guidelines to shift focus away from the recommendation to reduce saturated fat and toward recommendations to avoid added sugars.

Conversely, in a 2012 study, researchers evaluated the effects of a high saturated fat, low carbohydrate diet on the LDL patterns in healthy men. Following the diet, the group fed high amounts of saturated animal fat (in the form of beef fat) developed higher levels of healthy Pattern A LDL, with no increase in harmful Pattern B. The study also found that diets low in saturated fat and cholesterol are significantly associated with an increase in small, dense Pattern B LDL.

Multiple studies have corroborated these findings. Based on the research, it would seem the culprit is not saturated fat, but rather refined carbohydrates. Indeed, the LDL composition of a person consuming large amounts of saturated fat as their primary macronutrient is almost entirely pattern A. This is heart-protective!

But what about vegetable oils? The ones we were told to replace saturated fats with?

A 2018 Review on all of the available literature regarding omega-6 vegetable oil showed that oxidized LDL (Pattern B) actually comes from the oxidation of these vegetable oils contained within LDL. These polyunsaturated fats lead to harmful oxidized lipoproteins, which induce atherosclerosis and coronary heart disease. The researchers recommended *reducing* industrial vegetable oils for protection against heart disease. In a world which, across the board, is saying the exact *opposite*, these are brave and awesome scientists!

Over multiple studies, an increase in refined carbohydrates and Omega-6 Poly-unsaturated vegetable oils in the diet has been correlated with higher Pattern B LDL. Saturated fat, on the other hand, has only been shown to raise healthy Pattern A LDL. Think about what this means: we were told as a nation to cut out saturated fat and lower our total fat consumption. We were then instructed to replace saturated fat with Omega-6 vegetable oils. Instructions to lower dietary fat overall led to higher amounts of sugar in our foods. Both of these changes, done in the name of protecting us from heart disease, lead directly to Pattern B LDL. Pattern B LDL leads to heart disease. The irony is astounding!

LDL: Friend not Villain

It is well documented that both LDL and total cholesterol increase on a low carbohydrate diet. Likewise, LDL and total cholesterol increase during fasting. But why? The reason is simple: your body is metabolizing fat during low-carbohydrate dieting, as well as during fasting. As LDL is the molecule which delivers fatty acids throughout the body, of course it increases! It needs to deliver fat throughout your body to be burned away!

Scientists who despise both fasting and low-carbohydrate diets love to point out that these patterns of eating increase LDL, as well as total cholesterol. What has long perplexed them, however, is that simultaneously, the patients on a fasting or low carbohydrate diet also experience a reduction in triglycerides and insulin, with a simultaneous increase in HDL (good cholesterol). With the additional understanding of Pattern A versus Pattern B cholesterol, the picture comes into focus. While we are liberating fat from our bodies, LDL cholesterol does increase, but it is the healthy form of LDL which does so.

Contrast this to a diet rich in sugar, refined carbohydrates, and vegetable oil. Under the influence of this diet, LDL goes down. Fat is not being metabolized by the tissues but rather stored. The decrease in LDL is, therefore, due to a decreased need for fat metabolism, as glucose is the primary energy source. Despite this easily understood mechanism for reduced LDL on a highly refined carbohydrate diet, the scientists of the last few generations saw any reduction in LDL as beneficial. This simplification of complex metabolic science to "LDL is bad," has led to much of today's poor dietary advice.

While the dietary "experts" celebrated the lowering of LDL, they ignored the other important components of the lipid panel. On a diet rich in refined carbohydrates and sugar, despite the decrease in LDL, Triglycerides and insulin rise, and HDL (the good cholesterol) plummets. Simultaneously, the LDL, despite lower numbers, becomes comprised of almost all Pattern B LDL (or oxidized LDL). This is a very harmful and dangerous cholesterol panel!
LDL, then, has been unfairly vilified without proper understanding. Even today, for a physician to say LDL cholesterol may be **_good_** for the human body is close to medical **_heresy_**. Yet to those willing to look at the research, the benefits of Pattern A LDL are readily seen. Modern research is showing evidence that Pattern A LDL, as well as a diet rich in saturated fats, has amazing benefits.

Benefits of Pattern A LDL Cholesterol and Saturated Fat:

1. Immune function: Pattern A LDL cholesterol has been linked to lower rates of pneumonia and infection

2. Cancer Protection: Pattern A LDL cholesterol has been shown to reduce cancer rates

3. Heart Disease and Stroke: Pattern A LDL has been demonstrated to be cardioprotective, protecting against heart attack and stroke risk

4. Improved cognitive function: Pattern A LDL has been

shown to provide protection against Alzheimer's and Dementia

5. Antioxidant: Pattern A LDL upregulates antioxidant effects throughout the body. Similarly, it "soaks up" free radicals.

6. Apoptosis: Pattern A LDL increases autophagy and apoptosis of "Zombie" cells

7. Cell Repair: Pattern A LDL is vital to cellular repair and cell signaling

8. Co-Q10 Joint Protection: Pattern A LDL is vital to the delivery of Co-Q10 for maintenance of joint health

Stop Worrying

My point in presenting this research to you is to impress upon you something very important: our leading nutritional experts and advisors for the last 5 decades have chosen the wrong path. That much is clear — all of the evidence points in the opposite direction of their advice. The results of their influence are obesity, diabetes, heart disease, and stroke. Today we live in a world where someone truly believes eating factory-made chemical oil and sugar is protective of their heart!

Today many leading cardiologists, directly caring for patients with heart disease, are recommending a diet high in saturated fat and low in refined carbohydrates and vegetable oil. Rather than taking a cursory glance at someone's "LDL," these cutting-edge physicians are taking the necessary time to fully explore their patients' lipid panels and interpret them with common sense.

It is time for you to look around the world and see if the advice we have been given is working. Look at your coworkers, your family members, your spouse. Look at yourself. As a physician, I look around at my patients and my heart mourns. They are fat, diseased, sluggish, sad, and dying. And they have been told lies.

Do not, therefore, worry about saturated fat. Do not be suspicious of the food God made for you. Be suspicious of arrogant humanity, eager to replace foods we have eaten for millennia with their own abominations. Be suspicious of refined high-sugar carbohydrates and vegetable oils; of food made in a factory. These foods have done more to lead to heart disease than all of the saturated fat in the entirety of human history.

Rule #10: I will not fear saturated fat. Instead, I will fear chemical oils and sugar.

THE DR. CIMINO WEIGHT LOSS SOLUTION RULES

Rule #1: I will not eat any product with added sugar, nor will I eat any product with High Fructose Corn Syrup.

Rule # 2: I will not eat "Vegetable Oils" rich in Omega 6 fatty acids. When I need oil for cooking, I will use Olive Oil or Avocado Oil. When I cook with heat, I will simply use butter.

Rule #3: I will not eat refined carbohydrates. I will only eat carbohydrates which are naturally rich in fiber and minimally affect my blood glucose.

Rule #4: I will strive to keep my insulin levels at a minimum. This will allow glucagon to more easily become the dominant hormone, switching my body to fat metabolism.

Rule #5: I will strive to increase my sensitivity to Leptin. This will allow my body to "take inventory" of my fat stores, thereby decreasing my hunger and increasing my metabolism. To restore leptin sensitivity, I will first restore insulin sensitivity.

Rule #6: I will strive to make ketones my predominant body-fuel. I will not allow glucose and insulin to dominate my metabolism.

Rule #7: I will eat all of my calories in a 4-5-hour window. This will allow me to have maximal fat burning time throughout the rest of the day. It will allow me to reset my insulin resistance, increase leptin sensitivity, and escape the clutches of metabolic syndrome.

Rule# 8: Each day, I will begin my eating window with a large protein bolus. When possible, I will eat red meat to increase my carnitine levels.

Rule #9: I will eat a low-carbohydrate diet. Of this diet, I will eat as much as I want, without calorie counting. Likewise, I will not count macronutrient ratios. I will prefer protein over all other macronutrients.

Rule #10: I will not fear saturated fat. Instead, I will fear chemical oils and sugar.

CHAPTER 13: **ARTIFICIAL SWEETENERS**

Does Diet Soda Make You Fat?

Another of the most frequent questions I'm asked when discussing a diet designed to lower insulin and promote glucagon is: are artificial sweeteners ok? Most people, including myself, would love to be able to have a diet soda, or perhaps some sweetener in our black coffee during the hours in which we are not ingesting food.

The question, however, is a loaded one. To date, many trials have been conducted evaluating the effects of non-nutritive (or artificial) sweeteners on the body, and the results, though limited by sample size and study duration, have often been sensationalized by the media. After all, it makes a good headline, "Diet soda makes you fat!".

I remember working in the chemistry department in college, cheerfully drinking a diet coke, when a colleague of mine came up and said, "You know diet sodas make you fat, don't you? Just drink a regular soda." Of course, she did not know I was a type 1 diabetic, and could not drink regular soda, but still, her words have resounded in my head ever since. I held the can away from me. "Does this stuff make me fat?"

The Chicken or the Egg: Again!

Of interest to our study on weight loss, many trials have examined the role diet soda, and non-nutritive sweeteners (or artificial sweeteners as I refer to them) have had on obesity and metabolic syndrome (i.e., insulin resistance).

The majority of these studies purport to have found significant associations between artificial sweeteners and the development of metabolic diseases. But have they really?

Among these studies, a report from the Nurses' Health Study (NHS I and II) included more than 70,000 individuals. The study found a significant association between caffeinated artificially sweetened beverage consumption and the development of type 2 diabetes (insulin resistance). However, when the study was adjusted for energy intake and body mass (obesity), the association became statistically insignificant.

What this means is that due to the participants' obesity, body mass, and energy levels, the development of type 2 diabetes was statistically more likely to have stemmed from obesity itself, rather than from artificial sweeteners. The association to artificial sweeteners, therefore, becomes statistically insignificant. Yet the headline remained!

The Health Professionals Follow-Up Study evaluated the effects of Non-Nutritive Sweetener consumption on the development of type 2 diabetes. The study included approximately 40,000 male health professionals, whom it followed for over 20 years. Again, the study found a significant association between artificial sweeteners and the development of type 2 diabetes. But once again, this association was lost after an adjustment for obesity.

Finally, The European Prospective Investigation into Cancer and Nutrition (EPIC) Study, was a study performed in eight European countries. The study included 340,234 participants. This study reported a significant association between artificial sweeteners and type 2 diabetes development. But once again, the association lost its statistical significance after further adjustment for BMI and energy intake.

The problem, as you can see, is this: these studies are looking at obese individuals and then trying to sort out whether the diet soda is the cause of the development of diabetes over many years. Since obese individuals are the very ones who have trouble with blood sugar, this is truly trying to split hairs. To date, no conclusive evidence has been reported that shows non-nutritive sweeteners, in and of themselves, cause obesity or metabolic syndrome.

Artificial Sweeteners and the GI Tract

Does this mean that artificial sweeteners are ok? Not quite. As a substance not normally found in nature, it is important to realize that these chemicals were not intended for your body, but can serve, rather, as a possible crutch to aid in the reversal of insulin resistance. They should remain, at all times, suspect!

Among the possible harmful effects which have been studied, disruption of the gastrointestinal tract bacteria has shown some disturbing evidence.

A study done by Suez in 2014 demonstrated a change in the intestinal flora of participants who ate saccharin (the pink packet) for 7 days. These subjects, after 7 days on high amounts of saccharin, were experiencing higher blood glucose levels than prior to the study. Fascinatingly, after stool samples were taken from the study participants and placed in the GI tracts of mice, the mice also experienced increased blood glucose concentrations. This suggests that non-nutritive sweeteners affect the bacteria of the GI tract to a very large extent. As we have already discussed, this has the possibility of increasing whole-body inflammation, insulin resistance, insulin secretion, and obesity.

Some Studies Are Concerning

Likewise, some studies on non-nutritive sweeteners have shown a propensity for higher resting glucose levels and higher insulin levels. This is very interesting to our study on weight loss, as the last thing we want is to replace our eating style and diet, but yet increase our glucose and insulin through the substitution of artificial sweeteners.

A study done by Pepino in 2013 demonstrated increased glucose and insulin after a 7-day ingestion of large amounts of sucralose (commonly Splenda). Pepino also reported decreased insulin sensitivity as well as an increased serum insulin concentration. This is not good!

Looking at these studies, it appears we should run for the hills and never consider non-nutritive sweeteners again. But this is where things get complex. Despite the findings of the above studies, for every one study showing increased insulin or glucose, at least 10 other studies exist showing no effect whatsoever on glucose or insulin level.

A Look at the Studies:

A large, multi-study review completed in 2016 compared the effects of the major artificial sweeteners on insulin, blood glucose, and weight gain. The review noted differing and often contradictory results between all of the completed studies.

Listed below are the results:

Aspartame (Equal, blue packet): The review found 10 separate trials which showed aspartame does not raise blood glucose, insulin, or body weight. Only 1 study showed elevated glucose levels.

Sucralose (Splenda, yellow packet): The review found 8 high-quality studies which showed no influence on blood glucose, insulin, or body weight. 2 studies showed slightly elevated insulin levels.

Saccharin (Sweet n' Low, pink packet): The review found 2 high-quality studies showing no hormonal effects of saccharin. One study showed elevated glucose levels after 7 days.

Stevia (Green Packet): The review found 2 high-quality studies which showed no hormonal effect from Stevia. One study showed greater insulinogenic effect, meaning insulin levels went higher after carbohydrate consumption when in combination with Stevia. However, another study showed decreased insulin levels!

As you can see, the data are quite confusing. But there is at least a large cohort of data which does not show increased insulin resistance or increased glucose. But what about my own experience, as a type 1 diabetic, with these products?

In the name of science, I have embraced my own self-experimentation. Having tried all of the above sweeteners in large amounts, none has caused an increase in my blood glucose, nor an increase in my required insulin. This is encouraging and seems to fit with the above positive studies.

Don't Eat the Ones with Sugar

Unfortunately, even if the artificial sweeteners do not increase insulin or glucose concentrations in humans, we have another problem to deal with. Many of these products are packaged with sugar!

As a young diabetic, I was horrified to learn that the blue, pink, yellow, and green packets on most restaurant tables are 96% maltodextrin (sugar) and only 4% artificial sweetener. That's right! When you use any packet of non-nutritive sweetener, it has been packaged with 96% sugar to add bulk. Essentially you are just sweetening your coffee with sugar.

The powdered baking forms are no better. Today you must be careful to examine all powdered sweeteners, whether they be Stevia, Splenda, or any other. As you will find, in the large bags of these sweeteners intended for baking, most list maltodextrin as the primary ingredient. This essentially means you are using an alternative form of sugar, while erroneously thinking you are avoiding sugar.

The reason for this is simple. Most of these non-nutritive sweeteners are so sweet, a bag of 100% of them would be ridiculous. So, the companies need something they can bulk the product up with so that you are not buying a package the size of a raisin. They also want to have the baking instructions be similar to sugar. For this reason, they bulk the product.

To stay safe, use only the liquid versions of each product. In my home, we use liquid Splenda, liquid Stevia, and aspartame tablets. (None of which have added sugar)

Sugar Alcohols:

Besides the commonly used artificial sweetener, Sucralose (Splenda), Aspartame (NutraSweet), Stevia, Saccharin (Sweet and Low), some foods use "sugar alcohols" to sweeten their products. These sugar alcohols are chemically modified sugars.

Sugar Alcohols are typically much less sweet than normal sugar, and so are used in very high amounts. They are not digested by the GI tract, and therefore can be associated with abdominal cramping, flatulence, and diarrhea.

As a diabetic child, I ate an entire bag of gummy bears sweetened with these sugar alcohols, as the bag said they were "sugar-free". I had a regrettable night on the toilet, writhing in pain.

As sugar alcohols are becoming more popular in low carbohydrate diet recipes, I have listed the main ones below.

a.   Sorbitol is the primary sweetener used in chewing gum. It is typically created from dextrose that is derived from cornstarch. Sorbitol tastes 60 percent as sweet as regular sugar.

b.   Mannitol is made using fructose from cornstarch. Mannitol is 60 percent as sweet as regular sugar.

c.   Maltitol is made using maltose from cornstarch. It tastes 75 percent as sweet as regular sugar.

d.   Hydrogenated starch hydrolysates are made from cornstarch. Their sweetness is about 20 to 50 percent that of regular sugar.

e.   Erythritol is made from cornstarch. The process, unique among the sugar alcohols, involves fermentation. It tastes roughly 70 percent as sweet as sugar. Erythritol is gaining much popularity in recent years, and is used in many "Keto" recipes.

f.   Xylitol is often made from sugar cane. It is 95% as sweet as sugar. It also has a minty, cool taste, similar to menthol.

g.   Isomalt is made from sugar. It tastes roughly 55% as sweet as sugar.

h.   Lactitol is made from milk whey. Lactitol tastes 35 percent as sweet as regular sugar.

As you can see, all of these sugar alcohols are significantly less sweet than regular sugar. For this reason, they are used in double or triple the concentrations of regular sugar in baked goods. Beside gastrointestinal irritability, this leads to some other non-intended consequences. The main one is this: elevated blood glucose.

In the GI tract, the intestinal bacteria are able to convert these sugar alcohols into short-chain fatty acids which can then be absorbed by the GI tract. Sugar provides 6 calories per gram, and sugar alcohols 2-3 calories per gram. However, not all of these 2-3 calories come in the form of short-chain fatty acids. Some are re-converted into sugar.

In my own experimentation, all of the above sugar alcohols raise my blood glucose significantly. Erythritol, gaining popularity recently, is no different. Despite many people in the low-carb culture embracing erythritol, my own experience has been blood glucose elevations close to that of normal table sugar. That is true with all sugar alcohols. For this reason, I advise you to completely avoid sugar alcohols!

Sugar-Free Foods

Unfortunately, because of inadequate US food-labeling laws,

companies are permitted to label products "sugar-free" simply because they do not contain **table sugar**. The substitution, therefore, with another sugar has allowed companies to deceive consumers, including diabetics, into consuming these products and believing they are safe for someone trying to avoid sugar.

A great majority of the "sugar-free" products are full of ingredients which will substantially raise blood sugar, as well as insulin levels. These products, therefore, should be avoided when trying to heal insulin resistance, lose weight, or manage blood glucose (in diabetes).

Below is a list of the many deceptive ingredients placed in "sugar-free" foods which will raise your blood sugar substantially, and subsequently your insulin and weight:

Honey, Saccharose, Carob, Lactose, Sorbitol, Corn Syrup, Dextrin, Levulose, Sorghum, Dextrose, Treacle, Dulcitol, Maltodextrin, Maltose, Turbinado, Mannitol, Xylitol, Molasses, Glucose

What About Natural Sugar Alternatives?

Besides artificial sweeteners, I am also commonly asked about natural sugar substitutes, such as honey or Agave nectar. Honey is almost identical to table sugar chemically. It is a mix of glucose and fructose, which will quickly raise your blood sugar and insulin levels. One component makes it better than table sugar, however: in honey, there is a 20% wax and fiber component, which slows glucose absorption. While this is wonderful, it still raises blood sugar too quickly for the purposes of healing our insulin sensitivity.

Agave nectar, higher in fructose than sugar, should be avoided as well. In general, any caloric sweetener which can replace sugar in a recipe should be avoided, as it will raise blood sugar and insulin levels.

The Cimino Home

Since the data is so confusing, we must talk anecdotally. In the Cimino home, we use liquid Sucralose (Splenda) to sweeten our low carbohydrate chocolate, as well as our low carbohydrate cheesecake, and our morning coffee. We avoid all sweeteners which come in powdered form, as these are 96% sugar. We avoid honey, agave nectar, and any other natural sweetener which raises blood glucose and insulin.

I have never experienced increased blood sugar, with respect to my type 1 diabetes, after eating liquid Stevia, Splenda, or Aspartame. Likewise, I have never noted my insulin requirements to increase.

We do not fear diet soda sweetened with aspartame. I drink roughly 5-6 cans of aspartame-sweetened diet soda throughout the day. Is this good for my gut flora? Or my health in general? Probably not, but I share the information so that you can evaluate your own strategies when implementing the designs of the diet within this book.

During my fasting hours, I drink diet soda and have not noticed any decrease in ketosis. Likewise, I sweeten black coffee with liquid sucralose (Splenda), without any decrease in ketosis, rise in glucose level, or insulin requirement.

Similarly, my wife, after beginning this weight loss program, lost 45 pounds (from 167 pounds to 122 pounds), all while drinking aspartame-sweetened diet soda, and eating Splenda-sweetened chocolate (recipe in the back) like it was going out of fashion!

It is Your Choice

In the end, this must be your choice. The data are, at best, conflicted. Personally, I feel that if a little sucralose helps you avoid eating large amounts of regular sugar and worsening your spiral into insulin resistance and obesity, go for it! On the other hand, I respect a purist who wants nothing chemical added to their system. If that is you, likewise, do it! But there is not enough data to prove we should fear an insulin response from artificial sweeteners, and I personally have not found this to be the case.

Rules on sweeteners: Avoid artificial sweeteners in packet or powdered form, as these contain sugar. No sugar alcohols or "sugar-free foods" which contain the above ingredients. Avoid natural sugar replacements, such as honey or agave nectar. Check every artificial sweetener which you plan to use in recipes before buying. Many contain hidden maltodextrin or dextrose.

CHAPTER 14: ALCOHOL

Alcoholic Drinks

The next most frequently asked question I receive is: What about alcohol? Luckily, this is much easier to answer. Alcohol, in general, does not have profound effects on insulin or glucagon levels, except in the positive. Studies have shown that insulin sensitivity increases in the presence of alcohol. Likewise, glucagon levels increase. The data confirms this.

A 2015 meta-analysis showed alcohol consumption, in general, improved insulin sensitivity among women. Another study, performed in 2003, looked at heavy drinkers who considerably reduced their alcohol consumption, finding that a substantial reduction in alcohol intake from 7.2 to 0.8 standard drinks per day in healthy men did not change insulin sensitivity.

Other studies have reinforced either increased insulin sensitivity or have shown no change in insulin sensitivity. So, by and large, I have no issue with a person drinking the occasional alcoholic drink.

But this is where we need some caution. Most alcohol is not purely alcohol, but some combination of carbohydrate and alcohol. For example, a margarita contains a ton of sugar in the "Mix" before alcohol is even added.

Beer likewise can be very high in carbohydrate. Sweet Wine and Wine Coolers are almost always high in carbohydrate. The addition of carbohydrate will cause a glucose spike in your system, necessitating an insulin spike. This will lead to weight gain.

The Biochemistry of Ethanol

Within the body, ethanol is converted to acetyl-CoA. Acetyl-CoA can be used to generate glucose, amino acids, or fat. In individuals who have developed a beer belly, it is ***the combination of insulin*** with this ***precursor to fat***, derived from the breakdown of ethanol (alcohol), which leads to extra fat around the midsection. So, while alcohol is not prohibited, ethanol in combination with carbohydrate can quickly lead to fat storage.

In general, I recommend individuals stay away from alcohol while trying to lose weight, but I realize that not all will oblige this rule. The ideal use of alcohol during weight loss would be a small amount of dry wine with dinner. This is what I'd prefer you would drink if you just want to have a bit of alcohol each night.

Regardless of what you choose to do, for weight loss, try to observe two rules:

1.   Have your alcohol during your eating window. Preferably toward the end of your eating window.

2.   Secondly, drink only alcohol which is present in drinks with low amounts of carbohydrate. For example, dry wine rather than sweet wine. If you are fond of liquor, drink this with a diet soda or sugar-free seltzer.

Listed below are some of the common drinks in the United States and their carbohydrate content. Remember, a cup of regular corn-syrup sweetened soda contains about 25 grams of sugar. Use this as your basis of comparison.

Wine:

Dry Wine: 0.5 - 2 grams of carbohydrate per glass (minimal effect on glucose or insulin) -*Preferred*

Sweet Wine: 10 - 22 grams of carbohydrate per glass

Wine Cooler: 38 grams of carbohydrate

Beer:

Unfortunately, all beer is made from the fermentation of grain and is naturally high in carbohydrate. Avoid beer while trying to lose weight. If you must have beer, try to find an ultra-low carbohydrate version, but still, this is not advisable.

Within beer, there are examples of best to worst:

Light Lager (Low-Carbohydrate Beer): 4.9 grams of carbohydrate per bottle

Traditional Lager: 9.3 grams of carbohydrate per bottle

Ale: 15 grams of carbohydrate per bottle

IPA: 16 grams of carbohydrate per bottle

Malt Beverages: 32 grams of carbohydrate per bottle

Liquor:

Pure spirits such as vodka, gin, whiskey and tequila all have essentially 0 carbohydrates. By themselves, they should be fine on a low carbohydrate, insulin sensitivity diet. However, be careful not to mix with anything containing sugar! Use a sugar-free drink instead.

For example,

Rum and Coke: 36 grams of carbohydrate

Rum and Diet Coke: 0 grams of carbohydrate

Rule on Alcohol: When it comes to weight loss, the best idea is to simply avoid alcoholic beverages. This will result in the most rapid decline in body fat. If you must drink, do so at the end of your eating window and avoid carbohydrate-rich beverages.

CIMINO FAMILY RECIPES

In the following section, my wife, Jessica, has laid out many of the most common recipes which we eat as a family. She did an excellent job perfecting each recipe. I am now at the point where I beg like a child for her pot roast and jump with excitement when she tells me it is time for her Hibachi Chicken. She amazes me. I'm convinced she can find a way to make any recipe in a low-insulin form.

The recipes are laid out in the following sections: sauces and seasonings, meals, side dishes, and desserts. Because we have reclaimed saturated fat, eating delicious foods is not difficult to do on this program.

As well as the recipes in this book, please visit us at :

www.DoctorCimino.com

On our website, recipes will be continuously added. You can also send me any questions you may have, and I will try my best to answer them promptly. My goal is to see you succeed!

Also, feel free to search out low carbohydrate and ketogenic recipes online. If they follow the rules of this book, they are perfectly fine to use. Enjoy!

List of Recommended Items

As we will be making many of our own sauces, dressing, and desserts from scratch, we highly recommend the following cooking equipment:

1. Immersion Blender
2. Large Food Processor
3. Air Fryer
4. Wide Mouth Mason Jars & Reusable Lids
5. Squeeze Bottles
6. Electric Hand Mixer

Before the recipes…

Please leave us a review!

We truly hope you have found value in the content of this book. Our goal was to help to free you from the insulin-prison which has hurt so many lives in our time. We truly believe you will succeed if you follow the principles in this book.

If you have a spare moment, we would very much appreciate if you would review this book on Amazon. Reviews help prospective readers and are extremely valuable to our team!

Sauces and Dressings

Mayonnaise Base

(This will be the base for several dressing and sauces)

1 egg

3/4 cup avocado oil

1 teaspoon white vinegar

1 teaspoon lemon juice

1.   Start with a tall wide mouth mason jar.

2.   Add all ingredients and then pulse with an immersion blender for about 30-60 sec.

The egg and oil will emulsify to a thicker consistency the longer you blend them. You will see a thick, creamy, white mayonnaise form. This will make roughly 1 cup of your mayonnaise base. You can play around with amounts of each ingredient as you may prefer more vinegar flavor or less oil taste.

Warning: This recipe contains raw egg. Discuss with your doctor before consuming raw egg. We recommend pasteurized eggs, which have been pre-treated with heat to kill bacteria. We personally use "Davidson" brand.

Ranch Dressing

1 egg

3/4 cup avocado oil

1 tsp white vinegar

1 tsp lemon juice

1/2 tsp garlic powder

1/2 tsp onion powder

1 tsp dried parsley

1 tsp dried dill

1 tsp dried chives

1/2 tsp black pepper

1 tbsp water (add more water if you want thinner consistency)

salt to taste (avocado oil is already salty)

1.   Add all ingredients to a tall wide mouth jar and blend with an immersion blender until smooth.

This ranch is great on salads or as a dip for fried pickles.

Warning: This recipe contains raw egg. Discuss with your doctor before consuming raw egg. We recommend pasteurized eggs, which have been pre-treated with heat to kill bacteria. We personally use "Davidson" brand.

Greek Dressing

1 egg

3/4 cup olive oil

3 tbsp red wine vinegar

1 tbsp lemon juice

1-2 cloves minced garlic

1 tsp dried oregano

salt and pepper to taste

1.   Add all ingredients to a tall wide mouth jar and blend with an immersion blender until smooth.

This dressing is great for a Greek salad as well and on Mediterranean cauliflower rice or Mediterranean cucumber salad.

Warning: This recipe contains raw egg. Discuss with your doctor before consuming raw egg. We recommend pasteurized eggs, which have been pre-treated with heat to kill bacteria. We personally use "Davidson" brand.

Pink Sauce (for Hibachi Chicken)

1 cup Mayonnaise Base

1/2 tsp Garlic Powder

2 tsp Sugar-Free Ketchup

1/4 tsp Paprika

1/4 cup Water

2 tbsp Butter

1 "drop" Splenda liquid sweetener

1.　Start by melting your butter in the microwave for about 30 sec, or until completely melted.

2.　Create the Mayonnaise Base (see recipe above) and add in the garlic powder, ketchup, paprika, and water, then mix with a whisk until smooth.

3.　Next, add the melted butter. Mix with whisk.

4.　Add one "drop" of Splenda liquid sweetener. Use a measuring spoon to control how much is added, as this can make your sauce too sweet very easily. Mix with whisk.

Tzatziki Sauce

1 cup sour cream

1 tbsp lemon juice

1 tbsp dried dill

1/2 cup diced cucumber (peeled, with seeds removed)

1/4 tsp garlic powder

Salt to taste

1. Peel cucumber and dice.

2. Remove cucumber seeds and dice very fine.

3. In a large bowl, mix all ingredients together. Done!

Great as a veggie dip or with grilled Mediterranean chicken.

Seasoning Mixes

Basic Seasoning Mix

1/2 tsp salt

1/2 tsp pepper

1/2 tsp garlic powder

1/2 tsp onion powder

1/2 tsp paprika

1. Combine all ingredients together in a bowl.

Taco Seasoning

1 tbsp chili powder

1/2 tsp salt

3/4 tsp cumin

1/2 tsp dried oregano

1/4 tsp garlic powder

1/4 tsp onion powder

1. Add all ingredients in a large bowl and whisk together. You can save this in a jar as your standard taco seasoning (see taco bowl recipe below)

Chili Seasoning

2 tbsp chili powder

2 tbsp cumin

2 tsp paprika

1 tsp garlic powder

1 tsp onion powder

1 tsp dried oregano

1 tsp salt

pepper to taste

1/4 tsp cayenne pepper (optional for heat)

1. Add all ingredients to a large bowl and whisk together. You can save this in a jar as your standard chili seasoning (see chili recipe below)

Breading Mixture

1 cup parmesan cheese

1/2 tsp salt

1/2 tsp pepper

1/2 tsp garlic powder

1/2 tsp onion powder

1/2 tsp paprika

1.   Combine all ingredients together in a bowl and use as a breading to create fried pickles, zucchini, chicken, or anything else you would like to add "breading" before frying or air-frying.

Meals

Fool-Proof "Smashed" Burger

6 oz ground beef 80/20

salt and pepper to taste

Slice of cheddar cheese(optional)

1.   Weigh out 6 ounces of ground beef with a food scale. Gently form beef into a patty shape while trying not to over-handle the beef.

2.   Season with salt and pepper on both sides of the patty.

3.   Heat a frying pan on high heat. After it is fully heated, place the patty in the center and "smash" the patty as flat as you can with a spatula.

4.   Cook on this side for 3 min. After 3 minutes, flip burger and "smash" again. Cook for another 3 min on this side. You can add a slice of cheese at this point. (it will fully melt by the time your burger is done)

5.   Top with guacamole, goat cheese, bacon, or anything you like!

Enjoy! Our favorite way to serve this burger is with lettuce "wrap," dipped in ranch dressing or Pink Sauce. You may also serve with an "Egg Bread" hamburger bun (see recipe). A perfect side dish for this recipe is zucchini fries or fried pickles (see recipes).

Taco Bowl

1 lb. ground beef or turkey

1 tbsp olive oil

1/2 yellow onion chopped

1 chopped jalapeño pepper seeds removed (optional)

1 tbsp water

Taco seasoning mix (see recipe in seasonings section – seasoning recipe makes enough for 1 lb beef)

2 avocados diced into chunks

1/2 red onion chopped

2-3 Roma tomatoes seeds removed and diced

 1/2 cup shredded cheese (cheddar or Monterey jack)

1 tbsp olive oil

1 tbsp lemon juice

salt to taste

1.   Using a frying pan on medium heat, sauté the yellow onions, jalapeño, and ground beef or turkey in the olive oil until browned.

2.   Stir in the taco seasoning mixture. Add a small amount of water (1/4th cup) and stir, then set meat aside while you prepare the topping.

3.   In a large bowl, mix diced tomatoes, diced avocado, and red onion.

4.   Mix in lemon juice, olive oil, and cheese.

5.   Salt to taste.

6.   Serve taco meat on a bed of chopped lettuce and top with avocado mixture.

7.   Add sour cream if so inclined!

Excellent to serve or mix with Cauliflower Rice (see recipe)

"No Bean" Chili

1 lb. ground beef or turkey

1 tbsp olive oil

1 medium yellow onion chopped

1-2 cloves of garlic minced

1 cup diced carrots

1 14.5 oz can diced tomatoes (diced tomatoes are fine, pasta sauce is not!)

chili seasoning mix (see recipe in seasonings section – the recipe makes enough for one chili recipe)

2 cups water

sour cream and cheese for topping (optional)

1.   Brown meat in a pot with olive oil on medium heat.

2.   Add onions, carrots, and garlic to the pan, cooking until translucent.

3.   Add diced tomatoes, chili seasoning, and 2 cups water.

4.   Lower temperature to a simmer and cover.

5.   Let Chili cook for 30 min before serving.

6.   Top bowl of Chili with sour cream and shredded cheese (optional).

Classic Pot Roast

1 chuck roast

3-4 heads of garlic cut in half

1 tbsp dried thyme

Kosher salt

1 tsp black pepper

4-5 cups of water, depending on size of pot used

1.　　Preheat oven to 275-degree F.

2.　　Coat the outside of the roast in kosher salt and pepper.

3.　　Heat 2 tbsp of olive oil in a Dutch Oven (or cast-iron pot) on the stovetop. After oil is heated, sear roast, 30 sec on each side, or until golden colored. Be sure to sear the edges as well, using tongs to hold the roast in place.

4.　　After searing, set roast aside on a plate or cutting board. Slowly pour about 1 cup of water into the Dutch Oven while scraping any brown bits from the bottom of the Dutch Oven using a wooden spoon or spatula.

5.　　Add the roast back to the Dutch Oven. Add dried thyme, garlic halves, and enough water to almost cover the roast, then cover Dutch Oven with lid.

6.　　Move Dutch Oven to the regular oven and cook at 275-degrees for 5 hours, or until roast falls apart when stuck with a fork. You may need more time depending on the size of roast and oven type.

7.　　After removing roast, use a strainer to collect some of the juices to serve on the side as gravy.

8.   Serve with any side you like; we recommend a side salad and cauliflower mash. Pour gravy over roast. Enjoy small roast garlic chunks which have cooked alongside the roast!

Carolina Style BBQ Pork

For the Roast

1 bone-in Boston pork butt

4 tbsp. Salt

4 tbsp. Black Pepper

For the Sauce

1 cup apple cider vinegar

1/2 cup water

2 tbs red pepper flakes

1 tsp salt

1 tsp black pepper

1/4 tsp cayenne pepper (optional)

1.   You can make your sauce ahead the night before or right away. Just add all the sauce ingredients together in a jar, mix, and you're done. Set aside.

2.   For the roast preheat oven to 250-degree F.

3.   Rub the roast with salt and pepper.

4.   Line a roasting pan with tin foil and place roast fat side down.

5.   Move to oven and let cook for 2 hours per pound. Using a meat thermometer, look for a tempter of 195 degrees F in the center (Remember to start this early in the morning to allow plenty of cook time.)

6.   After removing the pork butt from the oven, allow to rest for one hour, covered by a dishtowel.

7.   Move pork to a large cutting board and chop with a large knife, then shred further with two forks.

8.   Make your sauce by combining all sauce ingredients in a bowl and stirring.

9.   Place meat in a large bowl or serving dish then toss with 1-2 tbsp of sauce. (Add as much as you like after tasting) You can serve the rest of the sauce on the side for dipping.

10.   Serve with coleslaw and fried zucchini, or make a sandwich with egg bread.

Margarita White Cauliflower Pizza

1/2 cauliflower

1 egg beaten

2 cups shredded mozzarella cheese

1 diced Roma tomatoes

dried basil

1 tsp olive oil + extra to drizzle on crust

1.   Preheat oven to 450 degrees F.

2.   Cut cauliflower into "bite-size" chunks. Using a food processer, chop cauliflower chunks until a grainy consistency.

3.   Place cauliflower into a kitchen towel and twist or squeeze to remove water. Try to get at least 1 tbsp of water out of the cauliflower. Look for a sand-like consistency of the cauliflower.

4.   Place cauliflower mixture into a large bowl and mix in beaten egg and 1 cup mozzarella cheese. You can also mix in 1 tsp garlic powder, 1 tsp onion powder, and some basil to make the crust more flavorful.

5.   Line a baking sheet with parchment paper and grease the center in a large circle by rubbing with olive oil.

6.   Place the cauliflower mixture onto the center of the greased parchment paper by pressing with your hands, forming

a large circle. You can try to press the edges in and build up a crust edge.

7.   Move to the oven and bake for 30 min or until your crust has a golden look.

8.   After the crust has baked, remove from the oven and let cool for 5 min.

9.   Drizzle remaining olive oil, then sprinkle on remaining cheese. Add diced Roma tomatoes and sprinkle with dried basil.

10.   Return to the oven to bake for 10-15 min or until cheese is fully melted. You can play with other seasoning or veggies; however, this is our favorite combination.

Fool-Proof Steak

New York strip steaks (as many as you'd like, or any other steak type)

1 box Kosher salt

2 cloves Minced garlic

2 tbsp. Butter

1.   Preheat oven to 275 degrees.

2.   Coat steaks in kosher salt. Do not be shy! Remember the edges!

3.   Line a baking sheet with aluminum foil, gently rub foil with olive oil.

4.   Place steaks on baking sheet and move to oven.

5.   Allow steaks to cook in oven for 25 minutes.

6.   After 25 minutes, remove from oven and move to frying pan. The frying pan should already be hot before removing steaks from oven. Put stovetop on maximum heat setting.

7.   Cook steaks 2 minutes on each side, and use tongs to sear the fatty edges for 1 minute each. (this will give all sides of your steak a nice brown color.

8.   Place garlic and 2 tbsp. of butter in a bowl. Microwave for 30 seconds, or until melted. Spoon this butter garlic mix over your steak.

9.   Let steak rest about 5 minutes. Enjoy!

If you prefer rarer meat, reduce oven time in 5-min increments.

Greek Chicken

2-3 chicken breast cut into cutlets

3 cloves minced garlic

1/4 cup olive oil, extra virgin

2 tbsp white wine vinegar

2 tbsp lemon juice

1 tbsp oregano, dried

1 tsp black pepper

1 tsp salt

1.   In a bowl combine garlic, olive oil, vinegar, lemon juice, oregano, salt, and pepper. This is your marinade mixture.

2.   Cut chicken into thin slices, cutting the chicken longways.

3.   Add the uncooked chicken to the marinade mixture and toss to make sure all the chicken is covered.

4.   Cover with plastic wrap and place in the refrigerator for a couple of hours. Marinating overnight will give even better flavor.

5.   When ready to cook, heat 1 tbsp olive oil in a pan on med heat. Add and cook chicken in batches to make sure each piece can make contact with the pan.

6.   Cook each batch of chicken until chicken is browned, about 3-4 minutes on each side.

7.   Serve with Tzatziki sauce (See Sauces Section), Cucumber Salad, and Mediterranean rice (Side Dishes).

Air Fryer Chicken Wings

6-8 chicken wings (if frozen, let thaw a couple of hours before cooking)

basic seasoning mix (See Seasoning Mixes)

1 tsp olive oil

1.   Set air fryer to 390 degrees F and allow to preheat for 5 min.

2.   Rub wings with basic seasoning mix.

3.   Most air fryers suggest lightly spraying with a cooking spray before cooking. You can either invest in a spray bottle filled with olive oil for this, or lightly drizzle about 1 teaspoon of olive oil over your chicken wings before placing them in the air fryer. Lightly oil chicken wings.

4.   Place wings in air fryer. Cook for 20 - 25 min. It is important to read your air fryers recommendations and cooking times as they may vary from brand to brand.

5.   Let wings cool for a few minutes before serving.

For Buffalo Wings

1 cup buffalo sauce or "hot sauce" (Find a brand with no added sugar!)

2 tbsp melted butter

Combine melted butter with buffalo sauce in a large bowl then toss with cooked chicken wings. Serve with ranch, celery, and carrots.

Chicken Salad

2-3 chicken breast

basic seasoning mix (See Seasoning Mixes)

¾ cup Mayo Base (add more or less to taste)

1/4 cup fine chopped celery

2 tsp dried dill

1/4 tsp poppy seeds

salt and pepper to taste

1 tbsp olive oil

leafy greens or thinly sliced pickles (optional to serve on)

1.   Preheat oven to 350 degrees F.

2.   Heat oil in a cast iron pot (or Dutch oven) on medium high heat. After pot is heated, add chicken breast and sear for 3-4 min on each side.

3.   After searing move the cast iron pot to the preheated oven and cook for 20 min.

4.   Remove chicken from cast iron pot.

5.   Allow cooked chicken to cool, then shred with two forks.

6.   Add all ingredients together in a bowl and serve on a bed of leafy greens or on thinly sliced pickles. If you are in

In Phase Two, you can add a few chopped almonds or walnuts for extra crunch.

Tuna Salad

1 can solid white albacore (packed in water)

3/4 cup mayo base

1/2 tbsp dried dill

salt and pepper to taste

leafy greens or thinly sliced pickles (optional to serve on)

1.   Drain water from turn can, pressing lid in to make sure max amount for water is removed.

2.   Add together all ingredients in a bowl and mix.

3.   Serve on leafy greens or thinly sliced pickles.

This is a great meal to take to work in a container!

Cauliflower Spinach Soup

1-pound beef or turkey

2 tbsp butter

1 cup onion diced

6 cloves minced garlic

1 head cauliflower chopped into chunks

12 oz package fresh spinach

3 cups water

1 cup Heavy Whipping Cream

1/2 cup shredded parmesan cheese

1.   In a large pan, brown ground beef (or ground turkey) with 1 tbsp butter, then remove and set aside.

2.   Add the second tbsp butter to the pan and sauté onions and garlic. Slowly pour 1/2 of water into the pot while scraping any brown bits with a wooden spoon or spatula. Add cooked meat, cauliflower, and rest of the water.

3.   Bring to a simmer and cover. Cook for 20-30 minutes or until the cauliflower is tender. Test with a fork, it should go through easily.

4.   Add the spinach and heavy whipping cream and continue cooking for 5-10 more minutes until spinach is cooked. Serve with fresh shredded parmesan cheese.

Broccoli Cheese Soup

1 lb. fresh broccoli (about 4 heads) chopped into small pieces

1 cup shredded carrots

1 diced onion

1/4 tsp nutmeg

1 - 8 Oz brick of cream cheese

8 oz shredded cheddar cheese

2 cups heavy whipping cream

1 tbsp butter

3 cups water

1.	Heat butter in a large cast iron pot (or Dutch Oven) on medium and sauté onions until lightly browned.

2.	Add in shredded carrots, chopped broccoli, and cream cheese. Stir cream cheese until melted.

3.	After cream cheese begins to melt, slowly add heavy whipping cream while whisking. Add water and nutmeg.

4.	Cover and let simmer for 15-20 minutes, until broccoli is tender. Do not bring to boil.

5.	Stir in shredded cheddar cheese. Once cheese is fully melted, about 5 minutes, serve.

Side Dishes

Cauliflower "Rice"

1 head cauliflower (depending on size of food processor)

1-2 tbsp butter

1 tsp garlic powder

salt and pepper to taste

1.   Chop cauliflower into small chunks.

2.   Using the "grater" disk on a food processor, shred the cauliflower to a "rice" like consistency.

3.   Heat butter in a large pan and sauté cauliflower until tender. As you Sautee, season with garlic, salt, and pepper.

4.   Experiment with any other seasonings you like, below are a couple of variations we like to make.

Mediterranean "Rice"

Add 1-2 tbsp Greek Dressing

1/4 cup kalamata olives (whole or sliced)

1/4 cup feta cheese

1/4 cup diced cucumber (peeled and deseeded)

1/4 cup sliced cherry/grape tomatoes

1/8 cup diced red onion

1.   Begin by making basic Cauliflower Rice (see recipe)

2.   In large bowl, add to rice: 1-2 tbsp Greek Dressing (see recipe), 1/4 cup kalamata olives (whole or sliced), 1/4 cup feta cheese, 1/4 cup diced cucumber (peeled and deseeded), 1/4 cup sliced cherry tomatoes, 1/8 cup diced red onion

Sautéed Spinach

10 oz. fresh spinach (1 bag)

1-2 tbsp olive oil

2-3 minced garlic

1 tbsp lemon juice

1/4 tsp salt

pepper to taste

1.	Heat oil in large pot over medium heat.

2.	Add garlic and sauté 1 minute or until garlic is aromatic but not brown.

3.	Add spinach, salt, and pepper and stir. As spinach begins to wilt, make sure to continue stirring. Cook about 4-5 mins.

4.	Remove from heat as soon as all the spinach has wilted down. Stir in lemon juice and season to taste if needed. Serve with a slotted spoon to help reduce moisture.

Oven Roasted Broccoli

2-3 head fresh broccoli

2-3 tbsp butter or lard

salt and pepper to taste

1.   Preheat oven to 450 degrees F.

2.   Line a baking sheet with parchment paper.

3.   Cut broccoli heads into 4ths, cutting in longways.

4.   Place the broccoli flat side down on the baking sheet. Cut butter or lard into equal chunks and place evenly across the tops of the broccoli. Season with salt and pepper then place in the oven.

5.   Bake for 15-20 minutes, or until broccoli is tender. Optional (Serve with shredded cheddar or parmesan cheese on top)

Egg Bread/Buns

3 eggs

3 ounces cream cheese

1.   Preheat oven to 300 degrees.

2.   Line a baking sheet with parchment paper (very important!)

3.   Separate egg yolks and whites into separate bowls.

4.   Using an electric hand mixer or stand mixer, whisk egg whites until firm, forming a meringue. About 5-6 minutes, until peaks form when you pull out the whisk.

5.   Mix the yokes and cream cheese. Combine the two mixtures by gently folding egg whites into the yolk mixture. Try not to stir too much.

6.   Scoop out "bun" size piles of egg mixture onto the parchment lined baking sheet. Try not make the piles too high. They should be about 4-inch diameter circles, 3/4 inches in height.

7.   Bake for 15-20 minutes or until golden on top. Let cool for 5 minutes. Use in place of a bun, or enjoy with melted butter.

Zucchini Fries

2-3 Zucchinis

breading mixture

2-3 eggs

1 tsp olive oil

1.   Use a wide dish to hold the Parmesan breading mixture (see recipe for breading). This will be used to coat the zucchini fries.

2.   Cut off zucchini ends and thinly slice zucchinis into "fry" size.

3.   Beat eggs in a bowl to coat the zucchini fries.

4.   One at a time, dip zucchini into the egg mixture (let excess egg drip off), and place in parmesan mixture. Be sure to make sure all sides are coated in the "breading."

5.   Using a paper towel, grease the fry basket of your air fryer by pouring the oil in and wiping out excess oil.

6.   Heat air fryer to 390 degrees. Let preheat for a few minutes.

7.   Add fries to the air fryer basket in batches so they are not crowded or on top of each other.

8.   Fry for 5-8 minutes, or until fries are golden and tender. (Tip, every 2-3 minutes remove the basket and toss the fries for better circulation)

9.   Enjoy with ranch dressing dip or sugar free ketchup.

Sour Cream and Chive Cauli-Mash (Substitute for Mashed Potatoes)

1 head cauliflower

1/2 cup water

1 tbsp butter

1/2 cup sour cream

1 tbsp dried chives

1 tsp salt

pepper to taste

1.   Chop cauliflower into small chunks.

2.   In a microwave safe bowl, heat cauliflower with water for 5-8 minutes or until cauliflower is tender.

3.   Test with a fork to easily pierce through. After cauliflower is fully cooked add butter to allow it to melt.

4.   Using an immersion blender, blend until cauliflower is "chunky".

5.   Add sour cream and continue to blend until smooth.

6.   Stir in salt, pepper, and chives.

Fried Pickles

2-3 large dill pickles

2-3 eggs

Parmesan "breading" mixture

1 tsp olive oil

1.   Use a wide dish to hold the Parmesan breading mixture (see recipe for breading). This will be used to coat the pickles.

2.   Cut pickles into 1/4-inch slices size. (Use whole pickles, as many pre-sliced pickles contain sugar)

3.   Beat eggs in a bowl.

4.   One at a time, dip pickles into the egg mixture (let excess egg drip off), and place in parmesan mixture. Be sure to make sure all sides are coated in the "breading."

5.   Using a paper towel, grease the fry basket of your air fryer by pouring the oil in and wiping out excess oil.

6.   Heat air fryer to 390 degrees. Let preheat for a few minutes.

7.   Add pickles to the air fryer basket in batches so they are not crowded or on top of each other.

8.   Fry for 5-8 minutes, or until fries are golden and tender. (Tip, every 2-3 minutes remove the basket and toss the fries for better circulation)

9.   Enjoy with ranch dressing dip.

Desserts

Coconut Chocolate (Our Favorite)

1 tbsp coconut oil

1 tbsp cocoa powder

1 tsp liquid Splenda

1 tbsp Shredded coconut (optional)

1/2 tsp vanilla extract

1.   Mix all ingredients together in a microwave safe bowl.

2.   Heat for 15-20 sec, or until oil is fully melted. Pour into silicone molds, or a parchment paper lined baking sheet.

3.   Place in freezer until solid, 30-60 min.

4.   After chocolate has frozen, remove from molds, or break into smaller pieces.

5.   Store in a freezer safe container, and keep in freezer. This chocolate will melt at room temperature and so is a frozen treat.

Naked Cheese Cake

3 Eggs, large

2 tsp liquid Splenda

2 tsp Vanilla extract, pure (optional swap out 1 tsp of vanilla for another flavor extract)

3 (8-oz.) blocks Cream cheese (tip, let get to room temp before starting cake)

2 cups Sour Cream

1 tbsp butter softened for greasing pan

1.   Preheat oven to 300°.

2.   Wrap the bottom of your 8" or 9" springform pan with parchment paper, then close the pan to lock the bottom in place. Cut away the excess parchment paper. Wrap the outside of the pan in tin foil to prevent leaks (this pan will sit in water).

3.   Using softened butter, grease the bottom and sides of the pan, and set aside.

4.   Place softened cream cheese in mixing bowl and whisk with electric hand mixer until lumps are gone.

5.   Add sour cream, vanilla, and sweetener. Whisk more until smooth, then taste for sweetness.

6.   Add more sweetener if you need to, then add eggs one at a time, fully mixing in each egg one at a time.

7.   Once mixture is completely smooth and free of lumps, spread evenly into pan.

8.   Place your foil-wrapped pan into a deep roasting pan. Fill up the roasting pan with boiling water until water reaches half-way up the springform pan.

9.   Bake for 1 hour 30 minutes. Turn off the oven and let the cake rest inside with the door slightly ajar for one hour.

10.   After cooling in the oven, you can remove cake from the water bath and remove the tin foil. Place in the fridge to allow to set for at least five hours, but preferably overnight.

Whipped Cream and Berries

1 cup heavy whipping cream

1 tsp vanilla extract

1 tsp liquid Splenda

berries of choice

1.   Pour whipping cream, vanilla, and Splenda into a tall wide mouth jar.

2.   Using an immersion blender, blend the cream until desired thickness, about 30-60 sec. The longer you blend, the thicker it becomes.

3.   Move to a bowl and eat with berries of choice. Strawberries, blackberries, raspberries, or blueberries. Or use as a topping.

Ice Cream

1 cup heavy whipping cream

1 tsp vanilla extract

1 tsp liquid Splenda

1 tsp flavor extract (orange, raspberry, caramel, lemon, any you like!)

Half cup of berries (if desired)

1.   Pour whipping cream, vanilla, flavor extract, and Splenda into a tall wide mouth jar.

2.   Mix in any desired berries. Using an immersion blender, blend the cream until desired thickness, about 30-60 sec. The longer you blend, the thicker it becomes.

3.   Pour into a loaf pan and cover with plastic wrap.

4.   Press the plastic wrap against the cream mixture to keep air out.

5.   Place in the freezer to freeze for 2 hours.

6.   Scoop, eat and enjoy!

For more recipes, visit us at DoctorCimino.com!

ABOUT THE AUTHOR

Scott A. Cimino, MD is a Christian, a father, a husband, and a practicing emergency physician. He holds degrees from Georgetown University and the University of North Carolina in biochemistry, human physiology, and medicine. Dr. Cimino's passion is the endocrinology and hormonal metabolism of the human body. As a type 1 diabetic since the age of 9, Dr. Cimino has had an up close and personal view of the hormonal inner workings of the human system. Sometimes too up close! He currently resides in Texas with his wife and three daughters.

For more information, or for any questions, visit our website at DoctorCimino.com

REFERENCES

Chapter 2:
1.   Hales CM, Carroll MD, Fryar CD, Ogden CL. Prevalence of obesity among adults and youth: United States, 2015–2016. NCHS data brief, no 288. Hyattsville, MD: National Center for Health Statistics. 2017.
2.   Fryar CD, Carroll MD, Ogden CL. Prevalence of Overweight, Obesity, and Severe Obesity Among Adults Aged 20 and Over: United States, 1960–1962 Through 2015–2016. National Center for Health Statistics. 2016.
3.   National Health Statistics Report No. 122 Dec 20th 2018 Mean Body Weight, Height, Waist Circumference, and Body Mass Index Among Adults: United States, 1999–2000 Through 2015–2016 Cheryl D. Fryar, M.S.P.H., Deanna Kruszon-Moran, Sc.M., Qiuping Gu, M.D., and Cynthia L. Ogden, Ph.D
4.   Ogden CL, Fryar CD, Carroll MD, Flegal KM.. Mean body weight, height, and body mass index, United States 1960-2002. Adv Data. 2004 Oct 27;(347):1-17.
5.   Keys, A., Brožek, J., Henschel, A., Mickelsen, O., & Taylor, H. L. The Biology of Human Starvation. (2 Vols.). Oxford, England: Univ. of Minnesota Press. 1950
6.   Yang W, et al. Prevalence of diabetes among men and women in China.N Engl J Med. 2010 Mar 25;362(12):1090-101. doi: 10.1056/NEJMoa0908292.
7.   World Health Organization. (2018, October 23). Healthy Diet. Retrieved March 15, 2019, from https://www.who.int/news-room/fact-sheets/detail/healthy-diet
8.   GBD 2015 Obesity Collaborators, Health Effects of Overweight and Obesity in 195 Countries over 25 Years. Engl J Med. 2017 Jul 6;377(1):13-27. doi: 10.1056/NEJMoa1614362.
9.   Kim MK, et al. Normal Weight Obesity in Korean Adults. Clin Endocrinol. 2014;80:214-220.
10.   Franco LP, Morais CC, Cominetti C. Normal-weight obesity syndrome: Diagnosis, Prevalence, and Clinical Implications. Nutr Rev. 2016 Sep;74(9):558-70. doi: 10.1093/nutrit/nuw019.
11.   Kaur J. A comprehensive review on metabolic syndrome. Cardiol Res Pract. 2014;2014:943162. doi: 10.1155/2014/943162.
12.   Vague J. Sexual differentiation. A determinant factor of the forms of obesity. 1947. Obes Res. 1996 Mar;4(2):201-3.
13.   Reaven GM. Banting lecture 1988. Role of insulin resistance in human disease. Diabetes. 1988 Dec;37(12):1595-607. doi: 10.2337/diab.37.12.1595.
14.   Kaplan NM. The deadly quartet. Upper-body obesity, glucose intolerance, hypertriglyceridemia, and hypertension. Arch Intern Med. 1989 Jul;149(7):1514-20.
15.   Molodecky NA, Soon IS, Rabi DM, Ghali WA, Ferris M, Chernoff G, Benchimol EI, Panaccione R, Ghosh S, Barkema HW, Kaplan GG. Increasing incidence and prevalence of the inflammatory bowel diseases with time, based on

systematic review. Gastroenterology. 2012 Jan;142(1):46-54.e42; quiz e30. doi: 10.1053/j.gastro.2011.10.001.

16.   Harper JW, Zisman TL. Interaction of obesity and inflammatory bowel disease. World J Gastroenterol. 2016 Sep 21;22(35):7868-81. doi: 10.3748/wjg.v22.i35.7868.

17.   Adışen E, Uzun S, Erduran F, Gürer MA. Prevalence of smoking, alcohol consumption and metabolic syndrome in patients with psoriasis. An Bras Dermatol. 2018;93(2):205–211. doi:10.1590/abd1806-4841.20186168

18.   Humphreys JH, Verstappen SM, Mirjafari H, et al. Association of morbid obesity with disability in early inflammatory polyarthritis: results from the Norfolk Arthritis Register. Arthritis Care Res (Hoboken). 2013;65(1):122–126. doi:10.1002/acr.21722

19.   Koyanagi A, Stickley A, Garin N, et al. The association between obesity and back pain in nine countries: a cross-sectional study. BMC Public Health. 2015;15:123. Published 2015 Feb 11. doi:10.1186/s12889-015-1362-9

20.   Shechter A, St-Onge MP, Kuna ST, et al. Sleep architecture following a weight loss intervention in overweight and obese patients with obstructive sleep apnea and type 2 diabetes: relationship to apnea-hypopnea index. J Clin Sleep Med. 2014;10(11):1205–1211. Published 2014 Nov 15. doi:10.5664/jcsm.4202

21.   Wood, K. (2015, July 22). "I have seen so many funerals for such a small island": The astonishing story of Nauru, the tiny island nation with the world's highest rates of type 2 diabetes. Retrieved March 15, 2019, from https://www.diabetes.co.uk/in-depth/i-have-seen-so-many-funerals-for-such-a-small-island-the-astonishing-story-of-nauru-the-tiny-island-nation-with-the-worlds-highest-rates-of-type-2-diabetes/

22.   Rosenfield RL, Ehrmann DA. The Pathogenesis of Polycystic Ovary Syndrome (PCOS): The Hypothesis of PCOS as Functional Ovarian Hyperandrogenism Revisited. Endocr Rev. 2016;37(5):467–520. doi:10.1210/er.2015-1104

23.   David P. McCormick, Kwabena Sarpong, Lindsay Jordan, Laura A. Ray, Sunil Jain. Infant Obesity: Are We Ready to Make this Diagnosis? The Journal of Pediatrics, 2010; DOI: 10.1016/j.jpeds.2010.01.028

Chapter 3:

1.   Center for Disease Control. (2018, February 13). Losing Weight. Retrieved March 15, 2019, from https://www.cdc.gov/healthyweight/losing_weight/index.html

2.   Chang, S. (2015, July 20). Reach Your Goal Weight Your Way with the NIH Body Weight Planner and USDA's SuperTracker. Retrieved March 15, 2019, from https://www.usda.gov/media/blog/2015/07/20/reach-your-goal-weight-your-way-nih-body-weight-planner-and-usdas

3.   World Health Organization. (2018, October 23). Healthy Diet. Retrieved March 15, 2019, from https://www.who.int/news-room/fact-sheets/detail/healthy-diet

4.   Guth, E. (2014, September 3). Healthy Weight Loss. Retrieved March 15, 2019, from https://jamanetwork.com/journals/jama/fullarticle/1900513

5.   American Heart Association. (2019). Losing Weight. Retrieved March 15, 2019, from https://www.heart.org/en/healthy-living/healthy-eating/losing-weight

6.   Leibel RL, Rosenbaum M, Hirsch J. Changes in energy expenditure resulting from altered body weight. N Engl J Med. 1995 Mar 9;332(10):621-8. doi: 10.1056/NEJM199503093321001.

7.   Nymo S, Coutinho SR, Torgersen LH, et al. Timeline of changes in adaptive physiological responses, at the level of energy expenditure, with progressive weight loss. Br J Nutr. 2018;120(2):141–149. doi:10.1017/S0007114518000922

8.   Dulloo AG, Jacquet J. Adaptive reduction in basal metabolic rate in response to food deprivation in humans: a role for feedback signals from fat stores. Am J Clin Nutr. 1998 Sep;68(3):599-606. doi: 10.1093/ajcn/68.3.599.

9.   Maclean PS, Bergouignan A, Cornier MA, Jackman MR. Biology's response to dieting: the impetus for weight regain. Am J Physiol Regul Integr Comp Physiol. 2011 Sep;301(3):R581-600. doi: 10.1152/ajpregu.00755.2010.

10.   Lazzer S, Boirie Y, Montaurier C, Vernet J, Meyer M, Vermorel M. A weight reduction program preserves fat-free mass but not metabolic rate in obese adolescents. Obes Res. 2004 Feb;12(2):233-40. doi: 10.1038/oby.2004.30.

11.   Ballor DL, Harvey-Berino JR, Ades PA, Cryan J, Calles-Escandon J. Decrease in fat oxidation following a meal in weight-reduced individuals: a possible mechanism for weight recidivism. Metabolism. 1996 Feb;45(2):174-8.

12.   Rosenbaum M, Hirsch J, Gallagher DA, Leibel RL. Long-term persistence of adaptive thermogenesis in subjects who have maintained a reduced body weight. Am J Clin Nutr. 2008 Oct;88(4):906-12. doi: 10.1093/ajcn/88.4.906.

13.   MacLean PS, Higgins JA, Jackman MR, Johnson GC, Fleming-Elder BK, Wyatt HR, Melanson EL, Hill JO. Peripheral metabolic responses to prolonged weight reduction that promote rapid, efficient regain in obesity-prone rats. Am J Physiol Regul Integr Comp Physiol. 2006 Jun;290(6):R1577-88. doi: 10.1152/ajpregu.00810.2005.

14.   Sumithran P, Prendergast LA, Delbridge E, Purcell K, Shulkes A, Kriketos A, Proietto J. Long-term persistence of hormonal adaptations to weight loss. N Engl J Med. 2011 Oct 27;365(17):1597-604. doi: 10.1056/NEJMoa1105816.

15.   Bray GA, Gallagher TF Jr. Manifestations of hypothalamic obesity in man: a comprehensive investigation of eight patients and a reveiw of the literature. Medicine (Baltimore). 1975 Jul;54(4):301-30. doi: 10.1097/00005792-197507000-00002.

16.   Lustig RH. Hypothalamic obesity: causes, consequences, treatment. Pediatr Endocrinol Rev. 2008 Dec;6(2):220-7.

17.   Atkinson MA, Eisenbarth GS, Michels AW. Type 1 diabetes. Lancet. 2014;383(9911):69–82. doi:10.1016/S0140-6736(13)60591-7

18.   Prentice RL, et al. Low-fat dietary pattern and risk of invasive breast cancer: the Women's Health Initiative Randomized Controlled Dietary Modification Trial. JAMA. 2006 Feb 8;295(6):629-42. doi: 10.1001/jama.295.6.629. PubMed PMID: 16467232.

19.   Howard BV, Van Horn L, Hsia J, et al. Low-fat dietary pattern and risk of cardiovascular disease: The Women's Health Initiative Randomized Controlled Dietary Modification Trial. JAMA : Journal of the American Medical Association.

Feb 8 2006;295(6):655-666.
20.   Beresford SAA, Johnson KC, Ritenbaugh C, et al. Low-fat dietary pattern and risk of colorectal cancer: The Women's Health Initiative Randomized Controlled Dietary Modification Trial. JAMA: Journal of the American Medical Association. 2006;295(6):643-654.
21.   Look AHEAD Research Group, Wadden TA, West DS, et al. The Look AHEAD study: a description of the lifestyle intervention and the evidence supporting it [published correction appears in Obesity (Silver Spring). 2007 May;15(5):1339. Wadden, Thomas A [added]; West, Delia Smith [added]; Delahanty, Linda [added]; Jakicic, John [added]; Rejeski, Jack [added]; Williamson, Don [added]; Berkowitz, Robert I [added]; Kelley, David E [added]; Tomchee, Christine [added]; Hill, James O [added]; K]. Obesity (Silver Spring). 2006;14(5):737–752. doi:10.1038/oby.2006.84
22.   The Look AHEAD Research Group Look AHEAD (Action for Health in Diabetes): design and methods for a clinical trial of weight loss for the prevention of cardiovascular disease in type 2 diabetes. Controlled Clinical Trials. 2003;24:610–628.
23.   Effect of intensive blood-glucose control with metformin on complications in overweight patients with type 2 diabetes (UKPDS 34). UK Prospective Diabetes Study (UKPDS) Group. Lancet. 1998 Sep 12;352(9131):854-65.

Chapter 4:

1.   Bernadette P. Marriott, Nancy Cole, Ellen Lee, National Estimates of Dietary Fructose Intake Increased from 1977 to 2004 in the United States, The Journal of Nutrition, Volume 139, Issue 6, June 2009, Pages 1228S–1235S, https://doi.org/10.3945/jn.108.098277
2.   Database for the added sugars content of selected foods, release 1. Nutrient Data Laboratory, Beltsville Agricultural Research Center, Beltsville Human Nutrition Research Center USDA : Agricultural Research Service, USDA; 2006.
3.   Casey, J. P. (1977), High Fructose Corn Syrup. A Case History of Innovation. Starch/Stärke, 29: 196-204. doi:10.1002/star.19770290605
4.   Le Tellier, A. (2012, June 27). Blame Nixon for the obesity epidemic. Retrieved March 15, 2019, from https://www.latimes.com/opinion/la-xpm-2012-jun-27-la-ol-nixon-obesity-epidemic-corn-20120627-story.html
5.   Keys A. Coronary heart disease in seven countries. 1970. Nutrition. 1997 Mar;13(3):250-2; discussion 249, 253.
6.   Johnson RJ, Segal MS, Sautin Y, Nakagawa T, Feig DI, Kang DH, Gersch MS, Benner S, Sánchez-Lozada LG. Potential role of sugar (fructose) in the epidemic of hypertension, obesity and the metabolic syndrome, diabetes, kidney disease, and cardiovascular disease. Am J Clin Nutr. 2007 Oct;86(4):899-906. doi: 10.1093/ajcn/86.4.899. Review. PubMed PMID: 17921363.
7.   Taubes, G. (2002, July 7). What if It's All Been a Big Fat Lie? Retrieved March 15, 2019, from https://www.nytimes.com/2002/07/07/magazine/what-if-it-s-all-been-a-big-fat-lie.html

8.   Leslie, I. (2016, April 7). The Sugar Conspiracy. Retrieved March 15, 2019, from https://www.theguardian.com/society/2016/apr/07/the-sugar-conspiracy-robert-lustig-john-yudkin

9.   David Kritchevsky, History of Recommendations to the Public about Dietary Fat, The Journal of Nutrition, Volume 128, Issue 2, February 1998, Pages 449S–452S, https://doi.org/10.1093/jn/128.2.449S

10.   Teff KL, Elliott SS, Tschöp M, Kieffer TJ, Rader D, Heiman M, Townsend RR, Keim NL, D'Alessio D, Havel PJ. Dietary fructose reduces circulating insulin and leptin, attenuates postprandial suppression of ghrelin, and increases triglycerides in women. J Clin Endocrinol Metab. 2004 Jun;89(6):2963-72. doi: 10.1210/jc.2003-031855.

11.   Faeh D, Minehira K, Schwarz JM, Periasamy R, Park S, Tappy L. Effect of fructose overfeeding and fish oil administration on hepatic de novo lipogenesis and insulin sensitivity in healthy men. Diabetes. 2005 Jul;54(7):1907-13. doi: 10.2337/diabetes.54.7.1907.

12.   Stanhope KL, Havel PJ. Fructose consumption: potential mechanisms for its effects to increase visceral adiposity and induce dyslipidemia and insulin resistance. Curr Opin Lipidol. 2008;19(1):16–24. doi:10.1097/MOL.0b013e3282f2b24a

13.   Froesch ER. Disorders of fructose metabolism. J Clin Pathol Suppl (Assoc Clin Pathol). 1969;2:7–12.

14.   Stanhope KL, et al. Consuming fructose-sweetened, not glucose-sweetened, beverages increases visceral adiposity and lipids and decreases insulin sensitivity in overweight/obese humans. J Clin Invest. 2009 May;119(5):1322-34. doi: 10.1172/JCI37385. Epub 2009 Apr 20. PubMed PMID: 19381015; PubMed Central PMCID: PMC2673878.

15.   Cox CL, Stanhope KL, Schwarz JM, et al. Consumption of fructose-sweetened beverages for 10 weeks reduces net fat oxidation and energy expenditure in overweight/obese men and women. Eur J Clin Nutr. 2012;66(2):201–208. doi:10.1038/ejcn.2011.159

16.   Mastrocola R, Collino M, Rogazzo M, Medana C, Nigro D, Boccuzzi G, Aragno M. Advanced glycation end products promote hepatosteatosis by interfering with SCAP-SREBP pathway in fructose-drinking mice. Am J Physiol Gastrointest Liver Physiol. 2013 Sep 15;305(6):G398-407. doi: 10.1152/ajpgi.00450.2012.

17.   Teff KL, Elliott SS, Tschöp M, Kieffer TJ, Rader D, Heiman M, Townsend RR, Keim NL, D'Alessio D, Havel PJ. Dietary fructose reduces circulating insulin and leptin, attenuates postprandial suppression of ghrelin, and increases triglycerides in women. J Clin Endocrinol Metab. 2004 Jun;89(6):2963-72. doi: 10.1210/jc.2003-031855.

18.   Basciano H, Federico L, Adeli K. Fructose, insulin resistance, and metabolic dyslipidemia. Nutr Metab (Lond). 2005;2(1):5. Published 2005 Feb 21. doi:10.1186/1743-7075-2-5

19.   Duffey KJ, Popkin BM. High-fructose corn syrup: is this what's for dinner?. Am J Clin Nutr. 2008 Dec;88(6):1722S-1732S. doi: 10.3945/ajcn.2008.25825C.

20.   Bocarsly ME, Powell ES, Avena NM, Hoebel BG. High-fructose corn

syrup causes characteristics of obesity in rats: increased body weight, body fat and triglyceride levels. Pharmacol Biochem Behav. 2010;97(1):101–106. doi:10.1016/j.pbb.2010.02.012

Chapter 5:

1.   Harcombe Z, Baker JS, DiNicolantonio JJ, Grace F, Davies B. Evidence from randomised controlled trials does not support current dietary fat guidelines: a systematic review and meta-analysis. Open Heart. 2016;3(2):e000409. doi: 10.1136/openhrt-2016-000409.

2.   Leren P. The Oslo diet-heart study. Eleven-year report. Circulation. 1970 Nov;42(5):935-42.

3.   Multiple Risk Factor Intervention Trial: Risk Factor Changes and Mortality Results. JAMA. 1982;248(12):1465–1477. doi:10.1001/jama.1982.03330120023025

4.   Dayton S, et al. A Controlled Clinical Trial of a Diet High in Unsaturated Fat in Preventing Complications of Atherosclerosis. Circulation. 1969;40:II-1–II-63.

5.   A co-operative trial in the primary prevention of ischaemic heart disease using clofibrate. Report from the Committee of Principal Investigators. Br Heart J. 1978 Oct;40(10):1069-118. doi: 10.1136/hrt.40.10.1069.

6.   Patek AJ, Toth IG, Saunders MG, Castro GAM, Engel JJ. Alcohol and Dietary Factors in Cirrhosis: An Epidemiological Study of 304 Alcoholic Patients. Arch Intern Med. 1975;135(8):1053–1057. doi:10.1001/archinte.1975.00330080055008

7.   Neaton JD, Blackburn H, Jacobs D, Kuller L, Lee DJ, Sherwin R, Shih J, Stamler J, Wentworth D. Serum cholesterol level and mortality findings for men screened in the Multiple Risk Factor Intervention Trial. Multiple Risk Factor Intervention Trial Research Group. Arch Intern Med. 1992 Jul;152(7):1490-500. PubMed PMID: 1627030.

8.   Ramsden CE, Zamora D, Majchrzak-Hong S, Faurot KR, Broste SK, Frantz RP, Davis JM, Ringel A, Suchindran CM, Hibbeln JR. Re-evaluation of the traditional diet-heart hypothesis: analysis of recovered data from Minnesota Coronary Experiment (1968-73). BMJ. 2016 Apr 12;353:i1246. doi: 10.1136/bmj.i1246

9.   Ramsden CE, Zamora D, Leelarthaepin B, Majchrzak-Hong SF, Faurot KR, Suchindran CM, Ringel A, Davis JM. Use of dietary linoleic acid for secondary prevention of coronary heart disease and death: Evaluation of recovered data from the Sydney diet heart study and updated meta-analysis. BMJ. 2013;346:e8707.

10.   Alvheim AR, Torstensen BE, Lin YH, et al. Dietary linoleic acid elevates endogenous 2-arachidonoylglycerol and anandamide in Atlantic salmon (Salmo salar L.) and mice, and induces weight gain and inflammation in mice. Br J Nutr. 2013;109(8):1508–1517. doi:10.1017/S0007114512003364

11.   Marchix J, Choque B, Kouba M, Fautrel A, Catheline D, Legrand P. Excessive dietary linoleic acid induces proinflammatory markers in rats. J Nutr Biochem. 2015 Dec;26(12):1434-41. doi: 10.1016/j.jnutbio.2015.07.010.

12.   Jandacek RJ. Linoleic Acid: A Nutritional Quandary. Healthcare (Basel).

2017;5(2):25. Published 2017 May 20. doi:10.3390/healthcare5020025
13.   Simopoulos AP. The importance of the ratio of omega-6/omega-3 essential fatty acids. Biomed Pharmacother. 2002 Oct;56(8):365-79.
14.   O'Brien, Richard D., et al. "Cottonseed oil." Chapter 5 in Bailey's Industrial Oil and Fat Products, Volume 2: Edible Oil & Fat Products: Edible Oils. Editor, Fereidoon Shahidi. John Wiley and Sons, Inc 2005.
15.   W. W. Yothers. Cotton Seed Oil Soap as a Substitute for Whale Oil SoapJournal of Economic Entomology, Volume 8, Issue 2, 1 April 1915, Pages 298–299.
16.   Guyenet SJ, Carlson SE. Increase in adipose tissue linoleic acid of US adults in the last half century. Adv Nutr. 2015 Nov;6(6):660-4. doi: 10.3945/an.115.009944. Print 2015 Nov.
17.   Lardinois CK, Starich GH, Mazzaferri EL, DeLett A. Polyunsaturated fatty acids augment insulin secretion. J Am Coll Nutr. 1987 Dec;6(6):507-15.
18.   Daley C, et al. A review of fatty acid profiles and antioxidant content in grass-fed and grain-fed beef Nutr J. 2010; 9:10.
19.   DiNicolantonio JJ, O'Keefe JH. Omega-6 vegetable oils as a driver of coronary heart disease: the oxidized linoleic acid hypothesis. Open Heart. 2018;5(2):e000898. doi: 10.1136/openhrt-2018-000898.
20.   Mozaffarian D , Rimm EB , Herrington DM . Dietary fats, carbohydrate, and progression of coronary atherosclerosis in postmenopausal women. Am J Clin Nutr 2004;80:1175–84.doi:10.1093/ajcn/80.5.1175
21.   Bemelmans WJ , Broer J , Feskens EJ , et al . Effect of an increased intake of alpha-linolenic acid and group nutritional education on cardiovascular risk factors: the Mediterranean Alpha-Linolenic Enriched Groningen Dietary Intervention (MARGARIN) study. Am J Clin Nutr 2002;75:221–7.doi:10.1093/ajcn/75.2.221

Chapter 6:

1.   Lucas López R, Grande Burgos MJ, Gálvez A, Pérez Pulido R The human gastrointestinal tract and oral microbiota in inflammatory bowel disease: a state of the science review. APMIS. 2017 Jan; 125(1):3-10.
2.   Singh RK, Chang HW, Yan D, et al. Influence of diet on the gut microbiome and implications for human health. J Transl Med. 2017;15(1):73. Published 2017 Apr 8. doi:10.1186/s12967-017-1175-y
3.   Cotillard A, et al. Dietary intervention impact on gut microbial gene richness. Nature. 2013 Aug 29; 500(7464):585-8.
4.   Canfora EE, Jocken JW, Blaak EE. Short-chain fatty acids in control of body weight and insulin sensitivity. Nat Rev Endocrinol. 2015 Oct;11(10):577-91. doi: 10.1038/nrendo.2015.128.
5.   Chambers L, et al. Optimising foods for satiety. Trends in Food Science & Technology Volume 41, Issue 2, February 2015, Pages 149-160. https://doi.org/10.1016/j.tifs.2014.10.007
6.   Ohlsson B, Darwiche G, Roth B, Bengtsson M, Hoglund P (2017) High Fiber Fat and Protein Contents Lead to Increased Satiety Reduced Sweet Cravings and Decreased Gastrointestinal Symptoms Independently of Anthropometric

Hormonal and Metabolic Factors. J Diabetes Metab 8:733.

7.   Wang ZQ, Zuberi AR, Zhang XH, et al. Effects of dietary fibers on weight gain, carbohydrate metabolism, and gastric ghrelin gene expression in mice fed a high-fat diet. Metabolism. 2007;56(12):1635–1642.

8.   Bueno L, Praddaude F, Fioramonti J, Ruckebusch Y. Effect of dietary fiber on gastrointestinal motility and jejunal transit time in dogs. Gastroenterology. 1981 Apr;80(4):701-7.

9.   Wrick KL, Robertson JB, Van Soest PJ, Lewis BA, Rivers JM, Roe DA, Hackler LR. The influence of dietary fiber source on human intestinal transit and stool output. J Nutr. 1983 Aug;113(8):1464-79.

10.   Silva FM, Kramer CK, de Almeida JC, Steemburgo T, Gross JL, Azevedo MJ. Fiber intake and glycemic control in patients with type 2 diabetes mellitus: a systematic review with meta-analysis of randomized controlled trials. Nutr Rev. 2013 Dec;71(12):790-801. doi: 10.1111/nure.12076.

11.   Carvalho C, et al. Plasma glucose and insulin responses after consumption of breakfasts with different sources of soluble fiber in type 2 diabetes patients: a randomized crossover clinical trial, The American Journal of Clinical Nutrition, Volume 106, Issue 5, November 2017, Pages 1238–1245, https://doi.org/10.3945/ajcn.117.157263Schulze

12.   Schulze MB, Hoffmann K, Manson JE, et al. Dietary pattern, inflammation, and incidence of type 2 diabetes in women. Am J Clin Nutr. 2005;82(3):675–715. doi:10.1093/ajcn.82.3.675

13.   Shewry, P. Wheat. Journal of Experimental Botany, Vol. 60, No. 6, pp. 1537–1553, 2009 doi:10.1093/jxb/erp058

14.   Cooper R. Re-discovering ancient wheat varieties as functional foods. J Tradit Complement Med. 2015 Jul;5(3):138-43. doi: 10.1016/j.jtcme.2015.02.004. eCollection 2015 Jul.

15.   Cani PD, Amar J, Iglesias MA, Poggi M, Knauf C, Bastelica D, Neyrinck AM, Fava F, Tuohy KM, Chabo C, Waget A, Delmée E, Cousin B, Sulpice T, Chamontin B, Ferrières J, Tanti JF, Gibson GR, Casteilla L, Delzenne NM, Alessi MC, Burcelin R. Metabolic endotoxemia initiates obesity and insulin resistance. Diabetes. 2007 Jul;56(7):1761-72. doi: 10.2337/db06-1491.

16.   Cani PD, Bibiloni R, Knauf C, Waget A, Neyrinck AM, Delzenne NM, Burcelin R. Changes in gut microbiota control metabolic endotoxemia-induced inflammation in high-fat diet-induced obesity and diabetes in mice. Diabetes. 2008 Jun;57(6):1470-81. doi: 10.2337/db07-1403.

17.   Zhang R, Jiao J, Zhang W, et al. Effects of cereal fiber on leptin resistance and sensitivity in C57BL/6J mice fed a high-fat/cholesterol diet. Food Nutr Res. 2016;60:31690. Published 2016 Aug 16. doi:10.3402/fnr.v60.31690

Chapter 7:

1.   Weissman C. Nutrition in the intensive care unit. Crit Care. 1999;3(5):R67–R75. doi:10.1186/cc360

2.   Unger, R. Glucagon and the Insulin: Glucagon Ratio in Diabetes and Other Catabolic Illnesses. Diabetes Dec 1971, 20 (12) 834-838; DOI: 10.2337/diab.20.12.834

3.   Ohneda, Akira & Parada, Eugenio & M. Eisentraut, Anna & Unger, Roger. (1968). Characterization of response of circulating glucagon to intraduodenal and intravenous administration of amino acids. The Journal of clinical investigation. 47. 2305-22. 10.1172/JCI105916.

4.   Marliss EB, Aoki TT, Unger RH, Soeldner JS, Cahill GF Jr. Glucagon levels and metabolic effects in fasting man. J Clin Invest. 1970;49(12):2256–2270. doi:10.1172/JCI106445

5.   Intensive blood-glucose control with sulphonylureas or insulin compared with conventional treatment and risk of complications in patients with type 2 diabetes (UKPDS 33). UK Prospective Diabetes Study (UKPDS) Group. Lancet. 1998 Sep 12;352(9131):837-53.

6.   Influence of intensive diabetes treatment on body weight and composition of adults with type 1 diabetes in the Diabetes Control and Complications Trial. Diabetes Care. 2001 Oct;24(10):1711-21. doi: 10.2337/diacare.24.10.1711.

7.   Russell-Jones D, Khan R. Insulin-associated weight gain in diabetes-- causes, effects and coping strategies. Diabetes Obes Metab. 2007 Nov;9(6):799-812. doi: 10.1111/j.1463-1326.2006.00686.x.

8.   Hartman YAW, Jansen HJ, Hopman MTE, Tack CJ, Thijssen DHJ. Insulin-Associated Weight Gain in Type 2 Diabetes Is Associated With Increases in Sedentary Behavior. Diabetes Care. 2017 Sep;40(9):e120-e121. doi: 10.2337/dc17-0787.

9.   Yadgar-Yalda R, Colman PG, Fourlanos S, Wentworth JM. Factors associated with insulin-induced weight gain in an Australian type 2 diabetes outpatient clinic. Intern Med J. 2016 Jul;46(7):834-9. doi: 10.1111/imj.13122.

10.   Leibel RL, Rosenbaum M, Hirsch J. Changes in energy expenditure resulting from altered body weight. N Engl J Med. 1995 Mar 9;332(10):621-8. doi: 10.1056/NEJM199503093321001.

11.   Conway B, Miller RG, Costacou T, Fried L, Kelsey S, Evans RW, Orchard TJ. Temporal patterns in overweight and obesity in Type 1 diabetes. Diabet Med. 2010 Apr;27(4):398-404. doi: 10.1111/j.1464-5491.2010.02956.x.

12.   Center for Disease Control. (2019). Prediabetes: Your Chance to Prevent Type 2 Diabetes. Retrieved March 15, 2019, from https://www.cdc.gov/diabetes/basics/prediabetes.html

13.   Coghlan, A. (2001, August 8). Athletes may be increasingly abusing insulin. Retrieved March 15, 2019, from https://www.newscientist.com/article/dn1129-athletes-may-be-increasingly-abusing-insulin/

14.   Atkinson MA, Eisenbarth GS, Michels AW. Type 1 diabetes. Lancet. 2014;383(9911):69–82. doi:10.1016/S0140-6736(13)60591-7

15.   Wilcox G. Insulin and insulin resistance. Clin Biochem Rev. 2005;26(2):19–39.

16.   Kınık MF, Gönüllü FV, Vatansever Z, Karakaya I. Diabulimia, a Type I diabetes mellitus-specific eating disorder. Turk Pediatri Ars. 2017;52(1):46–49. Published 2017 Mar 1. doi:10.5152/TurkPediatriArs.2017.2366

17.   Johnson JL, Duick DS, Chui MA, Aldasouqi SA.   Identifying prediabetes using fasting insulin levels. Endocr Pract. 2010 Jan-Feb;16(1):47-52.

doi: 10.4158/EP09031.OR.
18.   Sagild U, Littauer J, Jespersen CS, Andersen S: Epidemiological studies in Greenland 1962–1964. I. Diabetes mellitus in Eskimos. Acta Med Scand 179:29–39, 1966
19.   Mouratoff GJ, Scott EM: Diabetes mellitus in Eskimos after a decade. JAMA 226:1345–1346,1973
20.   Ebbesson SO, Schraer CD, Risica PM, Adler AI, Ebbesson L, Mayer AM, Shubnikof EV, Yeh J, Go OT, Robbins DC: Diabetes and impaired glucose tolerance in three Alaskan Eskimo populations: the Alaska-Siberia Project. Diabetes Care 21:563–569, 1998
21.   U.S. Department of Health and Human Services Office of Minority Health. (2017, August 25). Obesity and American Indians/Alaska Natives. Retrieved March 15, 2019, from https://minorityhealth.hhs.gov/omh/content.aspx?lvl=3&lvlID=62&ID=6457
22.   National Research Council (US) Committee on Population; Sandefur GD, Rindfuss RR, Cohen B, editors. Changing Numbers, Changing Needs: American Indian Demography and Public Health. Washington (DC): National Academies Press (US); 1996. 12, Diabetes Mellitus in Native Americans: The Problem and Its Implications.
23.   Gregg E, et al. Trends in the Prevalence and Ratio of Diagnosed to Undiagnosed Diabetes According to Obesity Levels in the U.S. Diabetes Care Dec 2004, 27 (12) 2806-2812; DOI: 10.2337/diacare.27.12.2806

Chapter 8:

1.   Paz-Filho G, Mastronardi C, Delibasi T, Wong ML, Licinio J. Congenital leptin deficiency: diagnosis and effects of leptin replacement therapy. Arq Bras Endocrinol Metabol. 2010;54(8):690–697.
2.   King BM. The rise, fall, and resurrection of the ventromedial hypothalamus in the regulation of feeding behavior and body weight. Physiol Behav. 2006 Feb 28;87(2):221-44. doi: 10.1016/j.physbeh.2005.10.007.
3.   Heymsfield SB, Greenberg AS, Fujioka K, et al. Recombinant Leptin for Weight Loss in Obese and Lean Adults: A Randomized, Controlled, Dose-Escalation Trial. JAMA. 1999;282(16):1568–1575. doi:10.1001/jama.282.16.1568
4.   Rosenbaum M, Murphy EM, Heymsfield SB, Matthews DE, Leibel RL. Low dose leptin administration reverses effects of sustained weight-reduction on energy expenditure and circulating concentrations of thyroid hormones. J Clin Endocrinol Metab. 2002;87:2391–2394.
5.   Coleman DL. A historical perspective on leptin. Nat Med. 2010 Oct;16(10):1097-9. doi: 10.1038/nm1010-1097.
6.   Kelesidis T, Kelesidis I, Chou S, Mantzoros CS. Narrative review: the role of leptin in human physiology: emerging clinical applications. Ann Intern Med. 2010;152:93–100.
7.   Velloso LA. The hypothalamic control of feeding and thermogenesis: implications on the development of obesity. Arq Bras Endocrinol Metabol. 2006;50:165–76.
8.   Licinio J1, Ribeiro L, Busnello JV, Delibasi T, Thakur S, Elashoff RM,

Sharma A, Jardack PM, Depaoli AM, Wong ML. Effects of leptin replacement on macro- and micronutrient preferences. Int J Obes (Lond). 2007 Dec;31(12):1859-63.

9.   Harris RBS. Is leptin the parabiotic "satiety" factor? Past and present interpretations. Appetite (2013) 61:111–8.10.1016/j.appet.2012.08.006

10.   Zhang Y1, Scarpace PJ. The role of leptin in leptin resistance and obesity. Physiol Behav. 2006 Jun 30;88(3):249-56.

11.   Segal K, et al. Relationship Between Insulin Sensitivity and Plasma Leptin Concentration in Lean and Obese Men Diabetes 1996 Jul; 45(7): 988-991.

12.   Cani PD1, Amar J, Iglesias MA, Poggi M, Knauf C, Bastelica D, Neyrinck AM, Fava F, Tuohy KM, Chabo C, Waget A, Delmée E, Cousin B, Sulpice T, Chamontin B, Ferrières J, Tanti JF, Gibson GR, Casteilla L, Delzenne NM, Alessi MC, Burcelin R. Metabolic endotoxemia initiates obesity and insulin resistance. Diabetes. 2007 Jul;56(7):1761-72. Epub 2007 Apr 24.

13.   Hervey GR. The effects of lesions in the hypothalamus in parabiotic rats. J Physiol. 1959;145(2):336–352. doi:10.1113/jphysiol.1959.sp006145

14.   Cani PD1, Bibiloni R, Knauf C, Waget A, Neyrinck AM, Delzenne NM, Burcelin R. Changes in gut microbiota control metabolic endotoxemia-induced inflammation in high-fat diet-induced obesity and diabetes in mice. Diabetes. 2008 Jun;57(6):1470-81. doi: 10.2337/db07-1403.

15.   Zhang R, Jiao J, Zhang W, et al. Effects of cereal fiber on leptin resistance and sensitivity in C57BL/6J mice fed a high-fat/cholesterol diet. Food Nutr Res. 2016;60:31690. Published 2016 Aug 16. doi:10.3402/fnr.v60.31690

16.   Zhang Y, Proenca R, Maffei M, Barone M, Leopold L, Friedman JM. Positional cloning of the mouse obese gene and its human homologue. Nature. 1994 Dec 1;372(6505):425-32. doi: 10.1038/372425a0.

Chapter 9:

1.   Pietiläinen KH1, Saarni SE, Kaprio J, Rissanen A. Does dieting make you fat? A twin study.Int J Obes (Lond). 2012 Mar;36(3):456-64. doi: 10.1038/ijo.2011.160.

2.   Shimazu T, Hirschey MD, Newman J, et al. Suppression of oxidative stress by β-hydroxybutyrate, an endogenous histone deacetylase inhibitor. Science. 2013;339(6116):211–214. doi:10.1126/science.1227166

3.   Phinney SD, Bistrian BR, Evans WJ, Gervino E, Blackburn GL. The human metabolic response to chronic ketosis without caloric restriction: preservation of submaximal exercise capability with reduced carbohydrate oxidation. Metabolism. 1983 Aug;32(8):769-76.

4.   Gasior M, Rogawski MA, Hartman AL. Neuroprotective and disease-modifying effects of the ketogenic diet. Behav Pharmacol. 2006;17(5-6):431–439.

5.   Reger MA, Henderson ST, Hale C, Cholerton B, Baker LD, Watson GS, Hyde K, Chapman D, Craft S Effects of beta-hydroxybutyrate on cognition in memory-impaired adults. Neurobiol Aging. 2004 Mar;25(3):311-4.

6.   Gasior M, Rogawski MA, Hartman AL. Neuroprotective and disease-modifying effects of the ketogenic diet. Behav Pharmacol. 2006;17(5-6):431–439.

7.   Freeman JM, Vining EP, Pillas DJ, Pyzik PL, Casey JC, Kelly LM The

efficacy of the ketogenic diet-1998: a prospective evaluation of intervention in 150 children. Pediatrics. 1998 Dec; 102(6):1358-63.

8. Hemingway C, Freeman JM, Pillas DJ, Pyzik PLThe ketogenic diet: a 3- to 6-year follow-up of 150 children enrolled prospectively. Pediatrics. 2001 Oct; 108(4):898-905.

9. Marsh EB, Freeman JM, Kossoff EH, Vining EP, Rubenstein JE, Pyzik PL, Hemingway C The outcome of children with intractable seizures: a 3- to 6-year follow-up of 67 children who remained on the ketogenic diet less than one year Epilepsia. 2006 Feb; 47(2):425-30.

10. Hernandez AR, Hernandez CM, Campos K, et al. A Ketogenic Diet Improves Cognition and Has Biochemical Effects in Prefrontal Cortex That Are Dissociable From Hippocampus. Front Aging Neurosci. 2018;10:391. Published 2018 Dec 3. doi:10.3389/fnagi.2018.00391

11. Ari C, Kovács Z, Juhasz G, Murdun C, Goldhagen CR, Koutnik AP, Poff AM, Kesl SL, D'Agostino DP Exogenous Ketone Supplements Reduce Anxiety-Related Behavior in Sprague-Dawley and Wistar Albino Glaxo/Rijswijk Rats. Front Mol Neurosci. 2016; (9):137.

12. Sacks H, Symonds ME. Anatomical locations of human brown adipose tissue: functional relevance and implications in obesity and type 2 diabetes. Diabetes. 2013;62(6):1783–1790. doi:10.2337/db12-1430

13. Lidell ME. Brown Adipose Tissue in Human Infants. Handb Exp Pharmacol. 2019;251:107-123. doi: 10.1007/164_2018_118.

14. Klement RJ. Beneficial effects of ketogenic diets for cancer patients: a realist review with focus on evidence and confirmation. Med Oncol. 2017 Aug;34(8):132. doi: 10.1007/s12032-017-0991-5.

15. Zuccoli G, Marcello N, Pisanello A, Servadei F, Vaccaro S, Mukherjee P, Seyfried TN. Metabolic management of glioblastoma multiforme using standard therapy together with a restricted ketogenic diet: Case Report. Nutr Metab (Lond). 2010 Apr 22;7:33. doi: 10.1186/1743-7075-7-33.

16. Nebeling LC, Miraldi F, Shurin SB, Lerner E Effects of a ketogenic diet on tumor metabolism and nutritional status in pediatric oncology patients: two case reports. J Am Coll Nutr. 1995 Apr; 14(2):202-8.

17. Contiero P, Berrino F, Tagliabue G, et al. Fasting blood glucose and long-term prognosis of non-metastatic breast cancer: a cohort study. Breast Cancer Res Treat. 2013;138(3):951–959. doi:10.1007/s10549-013-2519-9.

18. Forsythe CE, Phinney SD, Fernandez ML, Quann EE, Wood RJ, Bibus DM, Kraemer WJ, Feinman RD, Volek JS. Comparison of low fat and low carbohydrate diets on circulating fatty acid composition and markers of inflammation. Lipids. 2008 Jan;43(1):65-77. Epub 2007 Nov 29.

19. Srivastava S, Baxa U, Niu G, Chen X, Veech RL. A ketogenic diet increases brown adipose tissue mitochondrial proteins and UCP1 levels in mice. 2013;65(1):58–66. doi:10.1002/iub.1102

20. Cahill GF Jr. Fuel metabolism in starvation. Annu Rev Nutr. 2006;26:1-22. doi: 10.1146/annurev.nutr.26.061505.111258.

21. Schwatka F. The Long Arctic Search. E. Stackpole, Ed., The Marine Historical Assoc, Mystic CT 1965

22. McClellan W, et al. Prolonged Meat Diets with a study of Kidney

Function and Ketosis. JBC 87:651, 1930

23.   Sacks H, Symonds ME. Anatomical locations of human brown adipose tissue: functional relevance and implications in obesity and type 2 diabetes. Diabetes. 2013;62(6):1783–1790. doi:10.2337/db12-1430

24.   Kern PA, Finlin BS, Zhu B, et al. The effects of temperature and seasons on subcutaneous white adipose tissue in humans: evidence for thermogenic gene induction. J Clin Endocrinol Metab. 2014;99(12):E2772–E2779. doi:10.1210/jc.2014-2440

25.   Wheless, J. W. (2008), History of the ketogenic diet. Epilepsia, 49: 3-5. doi:10.1111/j.1528-1167.2008.01821.x

26.   Lee RWY, Corley MJ, Pang A, et al. A modified ketogenic gluten-free diet with MCT improves behavior in children with autism spectrum disorder. Physiol Behav. 2018;188:205–211. doi:10.1016/j.physbeh.2018.02.006

27.   US Cancer Statistics Working Group . United States Cancer Statistics: 1999-2010 Incidence and Mortality Web-based Report. US Department of Health and Human Services, Centers for Disease Control and Prevention, National Cancer Institute; Atlanta: 2013.

28.   Giovannucci E, Harlan DM, Archer MC, et al. Diabetes and cancer: a consensus report. Diabetes Care. 2010;33(7):1674–1685. doi:10.2337/dc10-0666

29.   Vigneri P, Frasca F, Sciacca L, Pandini G, Vigneri R. Diabetes and cancer. Endocr Relat Cancer. 2009 Dec; 16(4):1103-23.

Chapter 10:

1.   Henry R, et al. Intensive Conventional Insulin Therapy for Type II Diabetes: Metabolic effects during a 6-mo outpatient trialDiabetes Care Jan 1993, 16 (1) 21-31; DOI: 10.2337/diacare.16.1.21

2.   Cahill GF. Fuel metabolism in starvation. Annu. Rev. Nutr. 2006. 26:1-22 doi 10.1146/annurev.nutr.26.061505.111258

3.   Anton SD, Moehl K, Donahoo WT, et al. Flipping the Metabolic Switch: Understanding and Applying the Health Benefits of Fasting. Obesity (Silver Spring). 2018;26(2):254–268. doi:10.1002/oby.22065

4.   Marliss EB, Aoki TT, Unger RH, Soeldner JS, Cahill GF Jr. Glucagon levels and metabolic effects in fasting man. J Clin Invest. 1970;49(12):2256–2270. doi:10.1172/JCI106445

5.   Ho KY, Veldhuis JD, Johnson ML, et al. Fasting enhances growth hormone secretion and amplifies the complex rhythms of growth hormone secretion in man. J Clin Invest. 1988;81(4):968–975. doi:10.1172/JCI113450

6.   Gill S, Panda S. A Smartphone App Reveals Erratic Diurnal Eating Patterns in Humans that Can Be Modulated for Health Benefits. Cell Metab. 2015 Nov 3;22(5):789-98. doi: 10.1016/j.cmet.2015.09.005.

7.   Ribeiro M, López de Figueroa P, Blanco FJ, Mendes AF, Caramés B. Insulin decreases autophagy and leads to cartilage degradation. Osteoarthritis Cartilage. 2016 Apr;24(4):731-9. doi: 10.1016/j.joca.2015.10.017.

8.   Liu HY, Han J, Cao SY, et al. Hepatic autophagy is suppressed in the presence of insulin resistance and hyperinsulinemia: inhibition of FoxO1-dependent expression of key autophagy genes by insulin. J Biol Chem.

2009;284(45):31484–31492. doi:10.1074/jbc.M109.033936

9.   Glick D, Barth S, Macleod KF. Autophagy: cellular and molecular mechanisms. J Pathol. 2010;221(1):3–12. doi:10.1002/path.2697

10.   Longo VD, Panda S. Fasting, Circadian Rhythms, and Time-Restricted Feeding in Healthy Lifespan. Cell Metab. 2016;23(6):1048–1059. doi:10.1016/j.cmet.2016.06.001

11.   Chaix A1, Lin T1, Le HD1, Chang MW2, Panda S3.Time-Restricted Feeding Prevents Obesity and Metabolic Syndrome in Mice Lacking a Circadian Clock.Cell Metab. 2019 Feb 5;29(2):303-319.e4. doi: 10.1016/j.cmet.2018.08.004.

12.   Hatori M, Vollmers C, Zarrinpar A, et al. Time-restricted feeding without reducing caloric intake prevents metabolic diseases in mice fed a high-fat diet. Cell Metab. 2012;15(6):848–860. doi:10.1016/j.cmet.2012.04.019

13.   Chaix A, Zarrinpar A, Miu P, Panda S. Time-restricted feeding is a preventative and therapeutic intervention against diverse nutritional challenges. Cell Metab. 2014 Dec 2;20(6):991-1005. doi: 10.1016/j.cmet.2014.11.001.

14.   Hatori M, Vollmers C, Zarrinpar A, DiTacchio L, Bushong EA, Gill S, Leblanc M, Chaix A, Joens M, Fitzpatrick JA, Ellisman MH, Panda S. Time-restricted feeding without reducing caloric intake prevents metabolic diseases in mice fed a high-fat diet. Cell Metab. 2012 Jun 6;15(6):848-60. doi: 10.1016/j.cmet.2012.04.019.

15.   Brandhorst S, et al. A Periodic Diet that Mimics Fasting Promotes Multi-System Regeneration, Enhanced Cognitive Performance, and Healthspan. Cell Metab. 2015 Jul 7;22(1):86-99. doi: 10.1016/j.cmet.2015.05.012.

16.   Gotthardt JD, Verpeut JL, Yeomans BL, et al. Intermittent Fasting Promotes Fat Loss With Lean Mass Retention, Increased Hypothalamic Norepinephrine Content, and Increased Neuropeptide Y Gene Expression in Diet-Induced Obese Male Mice. Endocrinology. 2016;157(2):679–691. doi:10.1210/en.2015-1622

17.   Nair KS, Woolf PD, Welle SL, Matthews DE. Leucine, glucose, and energy metabolism after 3 days of fasting in healthy human subjects. Am J Clin Nutr. 1987 Oct;46(4):557-62. doi: 10.1093/ajcn/46.4.557.

18.   Bhutani S, Klempel MC, Berger RA, Varady KA. Improvements in coronary heart disease risk indicators by alternate-day fasting involve adipose tissue modulations. Obesity (Silver Spring). 2010 Nov;18(11):2152-9. doi: 10.1038/oby.2010.54.

19.   Catenacci VA, et al. A randomized pilot study comparing zero-calorie alternate-day fasting to daily caloric restriction in adults with obesity. Obesity (Silver Spring). 2016 Sep;24(9):1874-83. doi: 10.1002/oby.21581

20.   Zauner C, Schneeweiss B, Kranz A, Madl C, Ratheiser K, Kramer L, Roth E, Schneider B, Lenz K. Resting energy expenditure in short-term starvation is increased as a result of an increase in serum norepinephrine. Am J Clin Nutr. 2000 Jun;71(6):1511-5.

21.   Stewart WK, Fleming LW. Features of a successful therapeutic fast of 382 days' duration. Postgrad Med J. 1973;49(569):203–209. doi:10.1136/pgmj.49.569.203

22.   Espelund, et al. Fasting Unmasks a Strong Inverse Association between Ghrelin and Cortisol in Serum: Studies in Obese and Normal-Weight Subjects. The

Journal of clinical endocrinology and metabolism. 90. 741-6. 10.1210/jc.2004-0604.
23.   Natalucci G1, Riedl S, Gleiss A, Zidek T, Frisch H. Spontaneous 24-h ghrelin secretion pattern in fasting subjects: maintenance of a meal-related pattern. Eur J Endocrinol. 2005 Jun;152(6):845-50.
24.   Jones, J. (2013, December 19). In U.S., 40% Get Less Than Recommended Amount of Sleep Hours of sleep similar to recent decades, but much lower than in 1942. Retrieved March 15, 2019, from https://news.gallup.com/poll/166553/less-recommended-amount-sleep.aspx
25.   Weitzman ED, Fukushima D, Nogeire C, Roffwarg H, Gallagher TF, Hellman L. Plasma epinephrine and norepinephrine concentrations of healthy humans associated with nighttime sleep and morning arousal. J Clin Endocrinol Metab. 1971 Jul; 33(1):14-22.
26.   Atiea JA1, Aslan SM, Owens DR, Luzio S.Early morning hyperglycaemia "dawn phenomenon" in non-insulin dependent diabetes mellitus (NIDDM): effects of cortisol suppression by metyrapone. Diabetes Res. 1990 Aug;14(4):181-5.
27.   Emily J Dhurandhar et al The effectiveness of breakfast recommendations on weight loss: a randomized controlled trial The American Journal of Clinical Nutrition, Volume 100, Issue 2, August 2014, Pages 507–513, https://doi.org/10.3945/ajcn.114.089573
28.   Arble DM, Bass J, Laposky AD, Vitaterna MH, Turek FW. Circadian timing of food intake contributes to weight gain. Obesity (Silver Spring). 2009 Nov; 17(11):2100-2

Chapter 11:

1.   Pooyandjoo M, Nouhi M, Shab-Bidar S, Djafarian K, Olyaeemanesh A. The effect of (L-)carnitine on weight loss in adults: a systematic review and meta-analysis of randomized controlled trials. Obes Rev. 2016 Oct;17(10):970-6. doi: 10.1111/obr.12436.
2.   Tipi-Akbas P, Arioz DT, Kanat-Pektas M, Koken T, Koken G, Yilmazer M. Lowered serum total L-carnitine levels are associated with obesity at term pregnancy. J Matern Fetal Neonatal Med. 2013 Oct;26(15):1479-83. doi: 10.3109/14767058.2013.789847.
3.   Banting, W. (1885). Letter on corpulence, addressed to the public. London: Harrison.
4.   FALTA, W., & Meyes, M. K. (1923). Endocrine Diseases, including their diagnosis and treatment ... Translated and edited by Milton K. Meyers ... Third edition, with supplementary notes by the editor, etc. J. & A. Churchill: London; York, Pa. printed.
5.   Rosalyn Yalow, Solomon Berson, 1965 Frayn, K.N. 2010. Metabolic Regulation: A Human Perspective. 3rd edition
6.   Frayn, K. N. (2013). Metabolic regulation a human perspective. Chichester: Wiley-Blackwell.
7.   Bruch, H. (1957). The importance of overweight. New York: Norton.
8.   Spock, B. (1946). The common sense book of baby and child care.: With illus. by Dorothea Fox. New York: Duell, Sloan and Pearce.
9.   MacKarness, R. (1970). Eat fat: Grow slim. N.Y.: Pocket Books.

10.   Greene, R. (1951). The practice of endocrinology. Published on behalf of The Practitioner.
11.   Vilhjalmur Stefansson. (1929). New York: Macmillan.
12.   Taller, H. (1961) Calories Don't Count. Simon & Schuster; 1st edition
13.   Jou, C. (2011, April 8). Counting Calories. Retrieved March 15, 2019, from https://www.sciencehistory.org/distillations/counting-calories

Chapter 12:

1.   Mente A, de Koning L, Shannon HS, Anand SS. A systematic review of the evidence supporting a causal link between dietary factors and coronary heart disease. Arch Intern Med. 2009 Apr 13;169(7):659-69. doi: 10.1001/archinternmed.2009.38.
2.   Siri-Tarino PW, Sun Q, Hu FB, Krauss RM. Meta-analysis of prospective cohort studies evaluating the association of saturated fat with cardiovascular disease. Am J Clin Nutr. 2010 Mar;91(3):535-46. doi: 10.3945/ajcn.2009.27725.
3.   Hooper L, Summerbell CD, Thompson R, Sills D, Roberts FG, Moore H, Davey Smith G. Reduced or modified dietary fat for preventing cardiovascular disease. Cochrane Database Syst Rev. 2011 Jul 6;(7):CD002137. doi: 10.1002/14651858.CD002137.pub2.
4.   de Souza RJ, Mente A, Maroleanu A, Cozma AI, Ha V, Kishibe T, Uleryk E, Budylowski P, Schünemann H, Beyene J, Anand SS. Intake of saturated and trans unsaturated fatty acids and risk of all cause mortality, cardiovascular disease, and type 2 diabetes: systematic review and meta-analysis of observational studies. BMJ. 2015 Aug 11;351:h3978. doi: 10.1136/bmj.h3978.
5.   Ramsden CE, Zamora D, Majchrzak-Hong S, Faurot KR, Broste SK, Frantz RP, Davis JM, Ringel A, Suchindran CM, Hibbeln JR. Re-evaluation of the traditional diet-heart hypothesis: analysis of recovered data from Minnesota Coronary Experiment (1968-73). BMJ. 2016 Apr 12;353:i1246. doi: 10.1136/bmj.i1246.
6.   Hamley S. The effect of replacing saturated fat with mostly n-6 polyunsaturated fat on coronary heart disease a meta-analysis of randomized controlled trials. Nutr J. 2017;16:30–30.
7.   López-Jaramillo P, Otero J, Camacho PA, Baldeón M, Fornasini M. Reevaluating nutrition as a risk factor for cardio-metabolic diseases. Colomb Med (Cali). 2018;49(2):175–181. Published 2018 Jun 30. doi:10.25100/cm.v49i2.3840
8.   Astrup A, Dyerberg J, Elwood P, et al. The role of reducing intakes of saturated fat in the prevention of cardiovascular disease: where does the evidence stand in 2010?. Am J Clin Nutr. 2011;93(4):684–688. doi:10.3945/ajcn.110.004622
9.   DiNicolantonio JJ, O'Keefe JH. Omega-6 vegetable oils as a driver of coronary heart disease: the oxidized linoleic acid hypothesis. Open Heart. 2018;5(2):e000898. doi: 10.1136/openhrt-2018-000898.
10.   Mozaffarian D , Rimm EB , Herrington DM . Dietary fats, carbohydrate, and progression of coronary atherosclerosis in postmenopausal women. Am J Clin Nutr 2004;80:1175–84.doi:10.1093/ajcn/80.5.1175
11.   Bemelmans WJ , Broer J , Feskens EJ , et al . Effect of an increased intake of alpha-linolenic acid and group nutritional education on cardiovascular risk

factors: the Mediterranean Alpha-Linolenic Enriched Groningen Dietary Intervention (MARGARIN) study. Am J Clin Nutr 2002;75:221–7.doi:10.1093/ajcn/75.2.221

12.   Christakis G , Rinzler SH , Archer M , et al . Effect of the anti-coronary club program on coronary heart disease. Risk-factor status. JAMA 1966;198:597–604.doi:10.1001/jama.1966.03110190079022

13.   Ramsden CE , Zamora D , Leelarthaepin B , et al . Use of dietary linoleic acid for secondary prevention of coronary heart disease and death: evaluation of recovered data from the Sydney Diet Heart Study and updated meta-analysis. BMJ 2013;346:e8707.doi:10.1136/bmj.e8707

14.   Leslie, I. (2016, April 7). The Sugar Conspiracy. Retrieved March 15, 2019, from https://www.theguardian.com/society/2016/apr/07/the-sugar-conspiracy-robert-lustig-john-yudkin

15.   Harcombe Z, Baker JS, DiNicolantonio JJ, Grace F, Davies B. Evidence from randomised controlled trials does not support current dietary fat guidelines: a systematic review and meta-analysis. Open Heart. 2016;3(2):e000409. doi: 10.1136/openhrt-2016-000409.

16.   DiNicolantonio JJ, Lucan SC, O'Keefe JH. The Evidence for Saturated Fat and for Sugar Related to Coronary Heart Disease. Prog Cardiovasc Dis. 2016;58(5):464–472. doi:10.1016/j.pcad.2015.11.006

17.   Griffin BA1, Freeman DJ, Tait GW, Thomson J, Caslake MJ, Packard CJ, Shepherd J.Role of plasma triglyceride in the regulation of plasma low density lipoprotein (LDL) subfractions: relative contribution of small, dense LDL to coronary heart disease risk.Atherosclerosis. 1994 Apr;106(2):241-53.

18.   Berneis K. K., Krauss R. M. Metabolic origins and clinical significance of LDL heterogeneity. Journal of Lipid Research. 2002;43(9):1363–1379. doi: 10.1194/jlr.R200004-JLR200.

19.   Krauss RM Lipoprotein subfractions and cardiovascular disease risk. Curr Opin Lipidol. 2010 Aug; 21(4):305-11.

20.   Austin MA, Breslow JL, Hennekens CH, Buring JE, Willett WC, Krauss RM Low-density lipoprotein subclass patterns and risk of myocardial infarction. JAMA. 1988 Oct 7; 260(13):1917-21

21.   Rizzo M, Berneis K The clinical relevance of low-density-lipoproteins size modulation by statins. Cardiovasc Drugs Ther. 2006 Jun; 20(3):205-17.

22.   Arai H, Kokubo Y, Watanabe M, Sawamura T, Ito Y, Minagawa A, Okamura T, Miyamato Y Small dense low-density lipoproteins cholesterol can predict incident cardiovascular disease in an urban Japanese cohort: the Suita study. J Atheroscler Thromb. 2013; 20(2):195-203.

23.   Tribble DL, Holl LG, Wood PD, Krauss RM. Variations in oxidative susceptibility among six low density lipoprotein subfractions of differing density and particle size. Atherosclerosis. 1992 Apr;93(3):189-99.

24.   Ivanova EA, Myasoedova VA, Melnichenko AA, Grechko AV, Orekhov AN. Small Dense Low-Density Lipoprotein as Biomarker for Atherosclerotic Diseases. Oxid Med Cell Longev. 2017;2017:1273042. doi:10.1155/2017/1273042

25.   Faghihnia N, Mangravite LM, Chiu S, Bergeron N, Krauss RM. Effects of dietary saturated fat on LDL subclasses and apolipoprotein CIII in men. Eur J Clin Nutr. 2012;66(11):1229–1233. doi:10.1038/ejcn.2012.118

26. Campos H, Blijlevens E, McNamara JR, Ordovas JM, Posner BM, Wilson PW, Castelli WP, Schaefer E. LDL particle size distribution. Results from the Framingham Offspring Study. J.Arterioscler Thromb. 1992 Dec;12(12):1410-9.
27. Siri PW, Krauss RM. Influence of dietary carbohydrate and fat on LDL and HDL particle distributions. Curr Atheroscler Rep. 2005 Nov;7(6):455-9.
28. DiNicolantonio JJ, Lucan SC, O'Keefe JH. The Evidence for Saturated Fat and for Sugar Related to Coronary Heart Disease. Prog Cardiovasc Dis. 2016;58(5):464–472. doi:10.1016/j.pcad.2015.11.006
29. Siri-Tarino. Effects of diet on high-density lipoprotein cholesterol. Curr Atheroscler Rep. 2011 Dec;13(6):453-60. doi: 10.1007/s11883-011-0207-y.
30. U. Ravnskov, High cholesterol may protect against infections and atherosclerosis, QJM: An International Journal of Medicine, Volume 96, Issue 12, December 2003, Pages 927–934, https://doi.org/10.1093/qjmed/hcg150
31. Schultz BG, Patten DK, Berlau DJ. The role of statins in both cognitive impairment and protection against dementia: a tale of two mechanisms. Transl Neurodegener. 2018;7:5. Published 2018 Feb 27. doi:10.1186/s40035-018-0110-3
32. Zhou, F. High Low-Density Lipoprotein Cholesterol Inversely Relates to Dementia in Community-Dwelling Older Adults: The Shanghai Aging Study. Front Neurol., 12 November 2018. https://doi.org/10.3389/fneur.2018.00952
33. Valappil AV, Chaudhary NV, Praveenkumar R, Gopalakrishnan B, Girija AS. Low cholesterol as a risk factor for primary intracerebral hemorrhage: A case-control study. Ann Indian Acad Neurol. 2012;15(1):19–22. doi:10.4103/0972-2327.93270
34. Krauss RM Lipoprotein subfractions and cardiovascular disease risk. Curr Opin Lipidol. 2010 Aug; 21(4):305-11.
35. Diffenderfer MR, Schaefer EJ The composition and metabolism of large and small LDL. Curr Opin Lipidol. 2014 Jun; 25(3):221-6.
36. Ritenbaugh C, Patterson R, Chlebowski R, Caan B, Tinker L, Howard B, Ockene J. The WHI DM Trial: Overview and Baseline Characteristics of Participants. Ann Epidemiol 2003;13:S87-S97.
37. Prentice RL, Caan B, Chlebowski RT, et al. Low-fat dietary pattern and risk of invasive breast cancer: The Women's Health Initiative Randomized Controlled Dietary Modification Trial. JAMA : Journal of the American Medical Association. 2006;295(6):629-642.
38. Howard BV, Van Horn L, Hsia J, et al. Low-fat dietary pattern and risk of cardiovascular disease: The Women's Health Initiative Randomized Controlled Dietary Modification Trial. JAMA : Journal of the American Medical Association. Feb 8 2006;295(6):655-666.
39. Beresford SAA, Johnson KC, Ritenbaugh C, et al. Low-fat dietary pattern and risk of colorectal cancer: The Women's Health Initiative Randomized Controlled Dietary Modification Trial. JAMA: Journal of the American Medical Association. 2006;295(6):643-654.

Chapter 13:

1. Schulze MB, Manson JE, Ludwig DS, Colditz GA, Stampfer MJ, Willett WC, Hu FB. Sugar-sweetened beverages, weight gain, and incidence of type 2

diabetes in young and middle-aged women. JAMA. 2004 Aug 25; 292(8):927-34

2.   Romo-Romo A, Aguilar-Salinas CA, Brito-Córdova GX, Gómez Díaz RA, Vilchis Valentín D, Almeda-Valdes P. Effects of the Non-Nutritive Sweeteners on Glucose Metabolism and Appetite Regulating Hormones: Systematic Review of Observational Prospective Studies and Clinical Trials. PLoS One. 2016;11(8):e0161264. doi:10.1371/journal.pone.0161264

3.   Romaguera D, et al. Consumption of sweet beverages and type 2 diabetes incidence in European adults: results from EPIC-InterAct. Diabetologia. 2013 Jul; 56(7):1520-30.

4.   de Koning L, Malik VS, Rimm EB, Willett WC, Hu FB. Sugar-sweetened and artificially sweetened beverage consumption and risk of type 2 diabetes in men. Am J Clin Nutr. 2011 Jun; 93(6):1321-7.

5.   Pepino MY, Tiemann CD, Patterson BW, Wice BM, Klein Sucralose affects glycemic and hormonal responses to an oral glucose load. Diabetes Care. 2013 Sep; 36(9):2530-5.

6.   Suez J, Korem T, Zeevi D, Zilberman-Schapira G, Thaiss CA, Maza O, Israeli D, Zmora N, Gilad S, Weinberger A, Kuperman Y, Harmelin A, Kolodkin-Gal I, Shapiro H, Halpern Z, Segal E, Elinav E. Artificial sweeteners induce glucose intolerance by altering the gut microbiota. Nature. 2014 Oct 9; 514(7521):181-6.

7.   Holst JJ. The physiology of glucagon-like peptide 1. Physiol Rev. 2007 Oct;87(4):1409-39.

Chapter 14:

1.   Schrieks I, et al. The Effect of Alcohol Consumption on Insulin Sensitivity and Glycemic Status: A Systematic Review and Meta-analysis of Intervention Studies Diabetes Care 2015 Apr; 38(4): 723-732. https://doi.org/10.2337/dc14-1556

2.   Palmer JP, Ensinck JW.Stimulation of glucagon secretion by ethanol-induced hypoglycemia in man. Diabetes. 1975 Mar;24(3):295-300.

3.   Zilkens R, et al. The Effect of Alcohol Intake on Insulin Sensitivity in Men: A randomized controlled trial Diabetes Care 2003 Mar; 26(3): 608-612. https://doi.org/10.2337/diacare.26.3.608

Printed in Great Britain
by Amazon